TE DUE FOR RETURN

9

'99

01

⊦

__J5

Sexuality
and
Social Order

SEXUALITY
AND
SOCIAL ORDER

*The Debate over the Fertility
of Women and Workers in France,
1770—1920*

Angus McLaren

Holmes & Meier Publishers, Inc.
New York   •   London

First published in the United States of America 1983 by
Holmes & Meier Publishers, Inc.
30 Irving Place
New York, N.Y. 10003

Great Britain
Holmes & Meier Publishers, Ltd.
131 Trafalgar Road
Greenwich, London SE10 9TX

Book design by Rose Jacobowitz

Library of Congress Cataloging in Publication Data

McLaren, Angus.
  Sexuality and social order.

  Includes bibliographical references and index.
  1. Birth Control — France — History. 2. France — Social
conditions. 3. Robin, Paul. I. Title. [DNLM: 1. Family
planning — History — France. 2. Population control — History — France.   HQ 766.5.F8 M478s]
HQ766.5.F7M35   1983   304.6'6   81-13299
ISBN 0-8419-0744-7   AACR2

Manufactured in the United States of America

Contents

Preface

I would like to thank the following for their comments and suggestions:
Ralph Croizier, Anna Davin, Rod Day, Christine Delphy, Brian Dippie,
Chad Gaffield, Harvey Goldberg, John Gillis, Ruth Harris, John
Hutchinson, Ludmilla Jordanova, Tim LeGoff, Mary-Lynn McDougal,
Arlene Tigar McLaren, Pauline Marks, Harvey Mitchell, Matthew Ramsey,
David Stafford, Daniel Walkowitz, Judith Walkowitz, Theodore Zeldin and
the members of colloquia at St. Antony's College, Oxford, the History
Department at the University of California at Berkeley, the Davis Center for
Historical Studies at Princeton University, and the Women and Power
Conference at the University of Maryland. Special thanks to my typists
June Belton and Pat Cawley.

I was able to carry out the work on this study as a result of Faculty
Research Grants from the University of Victoria and a Canada-France
fellowship exchange program administered by the Social Sciences and
Humanities Research Council of Canada, for which I am greatly
appreciative.

Portions of this book have appeared in *Feminist Studies,* the *Journal
of the History of Ideas,* and *French Historical Studies*; I wish to thank the
editors and publishers for permission to reprint material which first
appeared in those volumes.

This book is for Jesse whose campaign to destroy the existing system
of sexuality and social order continues.

Sexuality
and
Social Order

Introduction

In 1920 the French Legislative Assembly, a body of men who had undoubtedly fathered fewer legitimate children than any other contemporary group of politicians, passed an act which endowed France with the most oppressive laws in Europe against contraception and abortion. Men who had themselves opted for small families thus legislated against the communication of information concerning the very practices they had so successfully employed. This staggering example of hypocrisy was but the culmination of a long defensive campaign against the propagation of birth control ideas in France, ideas most frequently associated in the public's mind at the turn of the century with the name of the libertarian Paul Robin. Robin, having committed suicide in 1912, did not experience the force of the new legislation, but his followers were subjected to harassment and persecution; Eugène Humbert, the most prominent, was to die in prison during an air raid in World War II.

The French birth control movement launched by Robin was, as in most other European countries, an offshoot of the British Malthusian League established in 1877. In 1878 and 1879 Robin attempted to win to the neo-Malthusian cause his friends in the French anarchist and socialist parties; failing in his efforts to have such groups adopt his policies, he established his own Ligue de la régénération humaine in 1896. The emergence of the movement elicited an amazing degree of public hostility, not because limitation of family size was unknown in France, but because it had already been employed by increaing numbers of couples for over a century. For this reason fears of actual depopulation had been expressed in the 1850s and repeated with alarm verging on hysteria after the country's humiliating defeat in 1870 at the hands of a more youthful and populous Germany. Accordingly, Robin's Ligue was immediately met by the creation of a rival Alliance nationale pour l'accroissement de la population supported by powerful elements within the church and military. The Alliance realized its first ambitions when the large losses in French manpower during the First World War precipitated the passage in 1920 of the act which tightened up the law on abortion and prohibited the diffusion of contraceptive information. It could be said that the campaign for fertility control had thus been lost, but a glance at the figures marking the continued drop in French natality in the 1920s and 1930s reveals the meaninglessness of such a statement. The real interest of the debate over birth control lies not in the purported effectiveness of either the opponents or proponents of such practices in influencing the family strategies of the masses. Neo-Malthusians no doubt had some effect in aiding those already bent on limiting family size just as priests and populationists succeeded in dissuading others. To seek to determine with any great degree of precision the impact of ideology on individual motivation is an impossible task. But what the literature thrown up by the debate does reveal are the social and sexual preoccupations of the combatants. In what follows, the ways in which a wide variety of commentators specifically related the issues of sexuality and social order will be the theme to which we will repeatedly return.

There exists no scholarly study of this intensely interesting fertility debate that raged between French doctors and priests, socialists and economists, neo-Malthusians and pronatalists at the turn of the century. Nor has much attention been paid to the ways in which women and workers responded to the arguments of those who pontificated on the duty to reproduce. This study has as its purposes both to provide a history of the birth control controversy in France from 1770 to 1920 and to show how such an analysis provides fresh insights on questions of medical, political, social, and sexual power in a society during a period of social transition.

A demographic revolution took place in Europe between 1850 and 1950. The high birth and death rates characteristic of a premodern society were replaced by a new pattern of lower fertility and lower mortality. It was France that took the lead in this transition. In England the birth rate reached a peak of 35 births per thousand in 1862 – 1878, after which it began its decline. But in France the birth rate had already fallen to 33 per thousand in the first decades of the century and was to be reduced even further as the century wore on. Thus it was to France that Europeans and North Americans looked for both practical demonstrations of the possibility of family limitation and ideological justifications or condemnations of birth control measures.

The desire to control fertility, which had a long history in France, found expression in a wide variety of forms ranging from postponed marriage to contraception to abortion. Nowhere else in Europe were people so candid in balancing social needs against individual desires. Long before their foreign contemporaries, French men and women perceived an advantage in having fewer children and in seeking ways to control family size. From the last decades of the eighteenth century more and more French women produced fewer and fewer children. And this decline continued through the first half of the nineteenth century despite the failure of any socially respectable defender of birth control to appear. Indeed social leaders publicly condemned what they took to be a threat to France's political power. The first questions to be posed in this study are therefore those dealing with the social forces which led to a decline in fertility and the political and religious preoccupations which fired the hostility to family limitation. Part One provides an explanation of the "demographic transition," including a discussion of both the reasons why increasing numbers of French couples would seek to limit their fertility and the tactics that they could employ. This first chapter provides a background to Part Two, in which the public expressions of hostility to the employment of contraceptives from the late eighteenth to the mid-nineteenth century are analyzed. The stance adopted by the Catholic church is examined in chapter two, the views of doctors in chapter three, the attitudes of secular moralists in chapter four, and the opinions of socialists in chapter five.

Why does the response of the French left loom so large in this study? First, because population control was associated in the public's mind with the conservative doctrines of Malthus and therefore political and demographic questions were as a consequence inextricably entangled. Secondly, because when birth control finally did find public defenders in the latter half of the nineteenth century, it was in the ranks of the libertarian left. Why this was the case is explained in Part Three in chapter six by examining the career of Paul Robin — anarchist, educator, and pioneer birth controller — and in chapter seven by showing the ways in which anarchists and syndicalists participated in the neo-Malthusian movement. What were the results of this curious alliance? One of its unexpected consequences was that France produced a unique birth control campaign that offered a radical critique of both sexual and political power, calling for both the right to abortion and social revolution. In countries such as the United States and Britain the birth control movement was captured by middle-class reformers and philanthropists and turned to the purposes of social control. In France, however, birth control was presented as a weapon in the class struggle. Anarcho-syndicalists discussed sexual matters in union halls in scenes that were not to be replicated until the Sex-Pol experiments of Wilhelm Reich in the 1920s.

What was the response won by the birth control campaign? Part Four examines the social, economic, and cultural concerns of women and workers which determined the ways in which they responded to the call for the *grève de ventre* and *libre maternité*. Chapter eight analyzes the attitudes of the working-class family toward birth control, and chapters nine and ten look at the reactions of women — be they feminists or not — to such forms of limitation as abortion. The argument will be made that workers and women were not as passive as is often implied in the demographic literature; to understand why a fertility strategy was accepted or rejected requires an examination of a group's complete social situation.

In Part Five the arguments of those opposed to birth control in the twentieth century are presented. In the conservative press a rising tide of hysterical protest against race degeneration and decline crested with the outbreak of World War I. As an outgrowth of the fear of Germany's population superiority, the French government passed savage anti-birth control laws and the French movement was driven underground. In chapter eleven the success of the conservatives in having repressive laws passed is weighed against their failure to have any serious impact on the further reduction of the birth rate in the twentieth century.

What conclusions can be drawn from such a history of the ideology and practice of birth control in France? First, as both a social issue and social movement, birth control serves as a barometer of secularization in a society undergoing change. Second, because of its importance to women, the success of family limitation can perhaps tell us more about women's power or passivity than the access to the vote (achieved in France only after World War II). Third, adoption of family limitation tactics was not due to technological change but to new social needs. Fourth, birth control pitted doctors against patients and it was the latter who in this area were the real medical innovators. Finally, because family limitation was not a typical political issue, the ways in which French politicians responded to it permits one to gain a new view of France freed of the archetypical left-right division.

This new view of nineteenth-century French society will emerge in the following pages as sexual and social ideologies are linked up. To accomplish this requires asking not just who opposed or defended contraception, but how the social and cultural concerns of the different sectors of French society necessitated their adoption of particular stances on the issue at particular times. The question is a complicated one, for as Foucault and others have argued, the public debate of sexual matters in the nineteenth century is not fully intelligible if viewed in isolation; the elaboration by doctors and demographers of the new science of sexology was a manifestation of a more general concern to bring the most intimate areas of private life within the pale of public policy.[1] Old-fashioned moralists were thus far from being alone in protesting against the idea of women and workers seeking a greater degree of autonomy through the employment of contraceptives. Progressive-minded politicians and social scientists were even more vehement in their denunciations of such purported moral anarchy which might endanger the nation. Both camps opposed not so much birth control itself but rather the lack of social discipline which it symbolized. With the advantage of hindsight it is easy to discount both the hopes and fears of those who believed that restriction of fertility posed a real threat to sex and class domination; only an appreciation of the relationships of sexuality and social order in nineteenth-century France allows one to understand the assumptions upon which such views were based.[2]

PART ONE

The Context

CHAPTER ONE

The Demographic Transition

Before broaching the ideological debate fought by the French in the nineteenth century over the rights and wrongs of birth control, it is first necessary to locate the discussion in its social context by determining the extent of recourse to contraception and abortion. Did French parents actually desire to limit family size? For what reasons? If determined to restrict conceptions, did they have access to the necessary contraceptive information or material? And was the resulting family limitation undertaken on such a massive scale as to warrant the wide-ranging intellectual controversy which it engendered? To answer these questions we must first turn to the analyses offered by historical demographers.

The science of demography was an invention of the French, the term coined in 1855 by Achille Guillard in his important study *Eléments de statistique humaine ou démographie comparée*. The date was significant, for the 1850s marked the emergence of obsessive concerns voiced by a host of social commentators who were alarmed by France's faltering fertility rate. The first half of the nineteenth century had witnessed in France a flowering of interest in the Malthusian doctrine regarding the need of a nation to avoid rapid population growth; the second half saw a return of eighteenth-century populationist sentiments.[1] Typical was the stance adopted by Léonce de Lavergne; having previously applauded much of Malthus's work, he carried out an about-face in 1857 when he attributed the French fall in fertility to "shameful calculations of egoism" which the "selfish" rationalized by reference to the teachings of the English economist.[2]

The concern expressed by Léonce de Lavergne and others for France's declining natality was sparked by the national censuses of the mid-century which revealed that the birth rate was falling far faster than the death rate. The first general census of France was carried in the *Mémoires* or reports of the intendants in 1697–1699 but only from 1801 on were the first modern compilations made. The populationist bias of most eighteenth-century commentators on fertility was accordingly based not on any clear idea of birth and death ratios, but on mercantilist beliefs that a growing population was the necessary precondition for a prosperous state.[3] The mistaken conviction occasionally expressed in the 1700s that

9

the population was actually declining was in turn a consequence of reports of depressions in agriculture and industry. Differences of opinion were expressed on the ways in which population growth might best be assured — for example, "luxury" was hailed by Voltaire and Montesquieu as an engine of progress while Quesnay, Rousseau, and Mirabeau père condemned it as being responsible for restriction of family size — but no one seriously questioned the necessity of such growth. Mercantilists at the beginning of the century declared that the state clearly had to be interested in promoting growth because masses of cheap labor provided its best guarantee of wealth and power by stimulating industry in peacetime and by manning the navies and armies in times of war. Physiocrats and philosophes at the end of the century asserted in more humane terms that growth was to be pursued because it promoted the health and happiness of all.[4]

In the first half of the nineteenth century orthodox economists dropped their support for government attempts to induce increased fertility, in part because the new national censuses revealed that France, far from losing population, had enjoyed an unprecedented growth between 1750 and 1800, in part because of the popularization of Malthus's work. Believers in laissez-faire could, in any event, hardly credit the state with the ability of violating the iron laws of economics. Their assumption, which gained increased currency, was that population, depending as it did upon subsistence, could not be forced to expand; it could only naturally respond to its social and economic environment. All the state could do was to inform the masses that, if they wished to avoid poverty, they had to embrace thrift and foresight while abstaining from marriage. The decline in the fertility rate in the early 1800s could be taken as evidence that such counsels were being followed, and the fall was therefore viewed by many with complacency. Indeed, the slowing rate of growth in the nineteenth century was noted in some accounts in self-congratulatory tones as a sign of the nation's culture and maturity. Optimistic Malthusians such as Legoyt, Quetelet, and de Broca insisted that the shift was a "natural" phenomenon, that though the birth rate was down the actual number of births per year was up, that the decline was volitional and not evidence of decay, that the resulting older age composition of the population was more favorable to productivity, and that, given the fact that those countries with the greatest population growth were the very ones with the most rampant poverty, the prudence of the French had to be applauded.[5]

These arguments were to an extent self-serving and were not accepted by those opposed to the status quo (such as the socialists) who continued to hold that population growth was the best barometer of a nation's prosperity. Even conservative commentators had to express some concern at the thought that France's political might abroad could be imperiled by the continual decline of fertility. When in 1854 and 1855 deaths actually exceeded births, there was sufficient evidence for the anxious to raise the cry that France was being endangered by depopulation. Léonce de Lavergne concluded in articles appearing in the *Revue des deux mondes* in 1855 and 1857 that something was profoundly wrong. The emperor himself in 1867 expressed his concern at the problems posed by recruitment; in 1868 L.A. Prévost-Paradol in *La nouvelle France* warned that if the fertility decline went on it would jeopardize France's foreign policy, cripple her colonial mission and reduce her to playing the role of Athens to Germany's Rome.[6] The crushing defeat to which France was subjected by Germany in 1870 seemed to bear out the arguments of these Cassandras.

The population anxieties expressed in moderate tones in the 1850s and 1860s were replaced in the 1870s by hysterical soul-searchings. Why had the country weakened itself to such an extent that it had fallen prey to its traditional rival? A vast range of arguments advanced to answer this question shared only the common premise that the fall in births was a disaster. Some felt that all European nations were going through a period of transition; others believed that there existed a specific French problem; some argued that the causes were short-term and unnatural, others, that they were long-term and inescapable. The right saw the fall in fertility as a result of the decline of the family and religion, the rise of feminism, education, and urbanism, the growth of materialism, greed and selfishness, and the pursuit of luxury, pleasure, and elegance. The left took the fall to be a result of capitalism's destruction of the family, industrialism's undermining of the natural sex roles, and Catholicism's poisoning of morality.

French demographers were attempting in the latter half of the nineteenth century to make sense of what their twentieth-century counterparts would, with the benefit of hindsight, term the "demographic transition": that is, the shift of population development from a pattern of high birth rates and high death rates to one of low birth rates and low death rates. Across western Europe from the middle of the eighteenth century onward, death rates fell whereas birth rates remained at their traditionally high levels of approximately 40 births per thousand. The result was a remarkable spurt in population growth, which was only curbed a hundred years later when birth rates also began to fall, thereby returning the system to a state of equilibrium. France was a special case, however, for here birth rates also began to fall during the eighteenth century; by the 1850s her population growth was negligible while that of the German states surged forward. The depopulationist fears expressed by French commentators were understandable given the fact that France was unique in having a declining birth rate; moreover, there appeared to be no end in sight to the decline. It was possible for the frightened to extrapolate figures to prove that the French would eventually disappear altogether.

The main premise on which so many of the nineteenth-century demographic theories were built was that in the past fertility had been uncontrolled or at best subject only to "natural" restraints but in the 1800s couples were for a variety of motives turning to "artificial" methods of control. The sociologist Frédéric Le Play, for example, sketched out a picture of a preindustrial society of extended family households which enjoyed high fertility. It was the Revolution, he asserted, which undermined the social cohesion based on the power of the patriarch by introducing laws which required the equal division of inheritances among all children. The peasant, faced with the choice of either being forced to split up his farm among many children or to pass it on intact to a single heir, now opted for the latter tactic. The result was an increasingly individualistic, unstable, pessimistic society in which contraceptive calculations played a central role.[7] The real story of the decline in the birth rate was far more complicated. In essence, what the transition in fertility revealed was that first, the numbers of births had always been subject to a variety of traditional social controls, for example, postponement of marriage; second, in exceptional cases coitus interruptus and abortion were also employed to limit fertility and over time played an increasingly important role as other methods fell in disfavor; and third, contraceptive practices which had been almost unanimously condemned in the eighteenth century eventually won favor in the nineteenth century because they were now part of normal marital behavior.

How was family size "traditionally" controlled in western Europe? Among the first discoveries made by modern demographers was that in France kinship was not as important as once thought; households tended, at least in the north, to be small and uncomplicated; and couples had far fewer children than was to be biologically expected. Restriction of family size was a result of limitations on those who were allowed to marry, postponement of marriage until the couple was in their late twenties, and spacing of births by the married.[8] These three social means of fertility control were in turn complemented by high rates of infant mortality. Who did not marry? The celibacy rate was highest among the nobility, ranging from 17 to 27 percent; among the peasantry it ran from 8 to 15 percent.[9] Such abstinence was in part institutionalized by communal groupings of monks, nuns, priests, soldiers, domestics, seminarians, and pensioners. In the main, however, such high rates of abstinence had to be the result of individuals deciding to forgo marriage for the benefit of the family's interest. The fact that in France such widespread celibacy was also accompanied by surprisingly low rates of illegitimacy — between 1 and 4 percent of all births in the eighteenth century — provides further evidence of the extent of social controls on sexuality.[10] Those who married did so relatively late in life; in the eighteenth century grooms were on average twenty-eight years of age, brides twenty-five. This signified that even if the bride had only reached sexual maturity in her late teens, she still had sacrificed at least six or seven years of potential childbearing. And if most marriages began late, many were soon terminated by the premature death of one or the other spouse. Assuming that the couple did survive until the woman reached menopause, she could be expected to have a child every two to two and one-half years up to the age of forty. Marriage was traditionally postponed until a couple could be assured of a degree of economic security — ideally by the peasant inheriting his father's farm. The spacing of births every two to two and one-half years was similarly undertaken by the mother in the hope of assuring the health of herself and her offspring.[11] It would have been possible to have borne far larger numbers of children, but French women opted for "quality" instead of "quantity." How were the long intervals between births achieved? Contraception and abortion no doubt played a role, an issue to which we will return, but for most mothers in the eighteenth century the spacing of births was probably accomplished by insisting upon conjugal abstinence during extended nursing. Lactation, we now know, in itself provides the nursing mother with some margin of protection against a subsequent conception. The mother's concern, however, was as much with the protection of her suckling child as with her own protection against pregnancy. The only safe food for the infant was mother's milk. Should the mother become pregnant and her breasts dry up, her baby would have to be fed on pap and accordingly its chances of an early death would increase. The mother would therefore appeal to traditional taboos against intercourse during nursing as a means of defending the health of the existing infant.[12]

By a variety of social means French fertility was controlled, but nevertheless large numbers of children died each year. In the seventeenth century one-fourth perished before their first birthday and another one-fourth before the age of twenty. The older children usually fell during the winter when food stocks were low, the younger ones in the epidemics of summer that ravaged a population already weakened by famine. At the best of times a farming system, in which two-fifths of the land was left fallow and yields were low, produced a weakened peasantry, malformed because of lack of proteins and vitamins, and wretchedly housed. Disease followed death before which doctors were helpless. Those who sought safety from epidemics by fleeing the cities only succeeded in spreading contagion. France, along with the rest of western Europe, was accordingly subject to a rhythm of population growth in periods of good harvests and decline in times of bad.[13] The first to die were the weakest — the very young and the very old. The woman who bore eight children could expect to raise only four or five. The overall consequence was the achievement, at the price of untold suffering and deprivation, of population equilibrium.

In the latter half ot the eighteenth century this equilibrium was lost. Mortality rates began to fall. Smallpox, which before 1789 was responsible for one-third of all deaths of children between the ages of one and four, disappeared. The famines and plagues so common to the seventeenth century were absent in the last decades of the eighteenth. Two-thirds of the population instead of only one-half would now reach the age of twenty. France's population, which had grown slowly from nineteen million in 1700 to twenty-one million in 1750, leaped to twenty-eight million in 1800.[14] But it was also in these very years of unprecedented population growth that the fertility rate began to be curbed.[15] Fertility could be still called "natural" as long as there was no interference with procreation as such and the woman had another pregnancy as soon as it was physiologically possible. It was the apparent violation of such laws discovered by historical demographers that provides evidence of birth control in preindustrial France. Louis Henry noted first in Geneva in the seventeenth century and also in France in the eighteenth that the number of children born to a woman did not vary as it logically should have with the marriage age of the woman. Women who married early had roughly the same number of children as those who married late, which signified that the former were employing some means to prevent pregnancy once the desired number of offspring was achieved. Henry found that despite life expectancy increases and declines in infant mortality the Genevan bourgeoisie had 5.4 children for the period 1600–1649, 3.6 for 1650–1699, and 2.9 for 1700–1749. By the eighteenth century similar patterns were noted among the families of both the French court and country aristocracy. In Besançon the number of children per Parlementarian family fell from 6.8 in 1692 to 4.4 in 1771–1790. Even in the small village of Lourmarin the number fell from 4.9 in 1726–1755 to 4.2 in 1756–1785, to 3.9 in 1786–1815.[16]

Why did the French undertake the "artificial" limitation of family size at so early a date? This question remains the key problem to which generations of historians and demographers have devoted their attention. The purpose of this study is to examine not the fertility decline itself but the debate which it precipitated. Nevertheless, to place the debate in context it is necessary to sketch out the general lines of argument generated by the current crop of demographic historians while noting that none has as yet produced a completely satisfactory explanation.[17] The oldest explanation of the wide-scale employment of artificial methods of birth control relies on a model in which a decline in infant mortality encumbers a family with more surviving children than expected. The woman who bore eight children and who logically expected to raise only four now finds that six survive and so falls back on contraception as a defensive method. That is to say, an artificial means of fertility control is employed when the natural methods fail. The problem posed by the French data is that although mortality rates as a whole fell in the eighteenth century, infant mortality rates were to remain high until the nineteenth century.[18] Demographers have therefore fallen back on a second argument that it was not so much the numbers of children surviving as it was their "utility" which changed. In a modernizing society children cease to be viewed as supplies of cheap labor and instead become expensive educational investments. Hence the upper and middle classes, faced with rising costs of the care and education of their offspring, had real economic incentives to limit family size. The flaw in this theory is that it remains to be proven whether extra children would have been a real *economic* burden even to those large numbers of couples employing contraception by the last decades of the eighteenth century whose educational expenses were minimal.[19] A third and more interesting idea, associated with the writing of Philippe Ariès, is that the number of children were limited not because they were seen as a burden but rather because they were more highly valued.[20] The eighteenth century witnessed a growing interest taken by the middle and upper classes in the happiness and well-being of children, a happiness which could only be economically assured if their number were limited. This increased sensitivity and greater degree of emotional investment manifested itself in parents' desire not to heap their estate just on the eldest child but to benefit all their offspring, daughters included. The first step in such a humanitarian undertaking, however, would presumably have been some attempt at lowering the infant mortality rate, a rate which the French upper classes kept remarkably high by their practice of sending their children out to wet nurses. A fourth explanation for the early decline in the birth rate attributes it to the greater degree of sexual equality enjoyed by French women.[21] Before the fertility transition approximately 10 percent of mothers died during pregnancy or its resulting complications, and women logically enough had an interest in reducing their exposure to such risks. That French women "domesticated" their spouses by imposing on them the practice of coitus interruptus is quite likely, but it remains to be explained why other women in other countries did not have the same success.

Turning to more general social explanations, one comes to a fifth argument based on the French concern for social mobility and materialism. To follow this line of argument it should be presumed that those seeking mobility would cut back on the expense of children; in fact the data suggests that most of the couples who first restricted family size did so for the defensive purpose of maintaining the status quo. The more prosperous the area, the lower the fertility; the higher the rates of poverty and mortality, the higher the fertility. To clarify this problem a sixth explanation has been elaborated according to which the high fertility of the remoter départements is understandable since they were cut off from the impact of urbanization and industrialization. The latter two forces would be the cause of fertility decline because in the cities less child labor was needed, information on contraception was more readily available, the atmosphere was more secular, and aspirations were higher. The weaknesses of this explanation lies in the fact that though France was the first nation in western Europe to lower its birth rate it was among the last to undergo urbanization and industrialization. If the social forces behind the fertility fall are hard to pin down, should one turn to ideological factors? According to a seventh theory it was the liberation of sexuality from theological constraints, the accompanying growth of scientific and rationalistic beliefs, and the pursuit of pleasure which led to birth control. Sauvy and Flandrin assert that the aristocracy took the lead first by discovering the technology of birth control through the secrets of prostitutes — the employment of douches and condoms — which the aristocracy then employed in courtly love and finally in marriage, and secondly by providing a model of the benefits of the small family. Their behavior was in turn aped by those attempting to improve their own standards — especially those peasants fearful of the breakup of their farms among too many heirs.[22] This explanation appears somewhat contrived because first, rates of religious observance and fertility cannot be related; second, coitus interruptus, not mechanical forms of contraception, was the main method employed in lowering the birth rate; and third, no evidence exists of the upper classes instructing the lower about contraception. It is simpler to accept the precocity of upper-class contraceptive behavior by attributing it to a greater concern to protect inherited wealth on which economic stability depended, and to argue that the similar, later behavior of the lower classes was a case not of their "aping their betters" but of responding to their own social and economic concerns.

Clearly a whole constellation of social and ideological forces was involved in the peculiar fertility behavior of the French. If it continues to puzzle twentieth-century researchers, it is all the more understandable why it should have mystified commentators in the eighteenth and nineteenth centuries. The one thing that should be obvious from the above abbreviated discussion is that the employment of contraceptive techniques was not simply the replacement by artificial controls of the high rate of infant mortality as a means of limiting family size. All the old determinants of fertility underwent change.[23] Celibacy rates went down as more couples married than had in the past. The legalization of divorce and simplification of marriage formalities during the Revolution removed the legal barriers, while contraception removed potential economic barriers, that previously had prevented weddings. For the general population, age of marriage would remain in the mid-twenties right through the nineteenth century, but for the aristocracy it dropped dramatically as did the age at which the mother had her last child. Indeed, restriction of family size was matched by concentration of births. Whereas in the past births had been separated by long birth intervals and marked by the late age of the mother at the last pregnancy, in the nineteenth century the mother had her children earlier and in more rapid succession. Contraception was employed not to postpone family obligations but rather to end them. Thus the biggest drop in births took place among older women who employed techniques to stop further conceptions once the desired family size was achieved. Extended nursing, which was once used to space births, became less popular, and this in itself was an additional reason for recourse to contraception. Noblewomen in the eighteenth century who gave up breast-feeding because of a distaste for what was construed as an "animal" function found themselves losing a margin of contraceptive protection as well as an argument against resumption of their conjugal duties; if they wished to avoid a further pregnancy, contraception was the only answer. In the mid-nineteenth century, working women whose responsibilities forced them to send out their own children to be wet-nursed — in Paris close to two-thirds of the children were wet-nursed — faced the same problem.[24]

The debate over the cause of the artificial limitation of family size in France is far from being concluded, but the constellation of contributing forces has been well mapped out by historians. Clearly the increased concern for family privacy, the rise of affection of men for women, of parents for children (or at least the rise in public declarations of the desirability of such emotions), the increased costs of even the rudimentary education available in the eighteenth century, the ideological sanctions for family concerns offered by both Catholic theologians and rationalist philosophes, and the growth of individualism as a consequence of the expansion of the market economy all played a role. Accordingly, the restriction of fertility was presumably related to the views eighteenth- and nineteenth-century French men and women held about their ability to manipulate their environment. But how *new* were such attitudes? Some historians have argued that the French in limiting conceptions were making a distinction between reproduction and pleasure and thereby providing a manifestation of what has been called the emerging "modern personality";

others have suggested that such actions were simply a consequence of France's unique dedication to small proprietorship. A review of the methods employed by the French provides some insights into the originality of their contraceptive behavior.

How did French couples reduce the number of births? The French experience of a declining fertility rate does not fit the simple model of birth control being a consequence, on the one hand, of a falling infant mortality rate and, on the other, the availability of new contraceptive information. Infant mortality rates remained high and the largely illiterate population of a still overwhelmingly rural country was cut off from sophisticated, urban, birth control techniques. Some historians and demographers continue to insist that without access to such information the mass reduction of fertility is impossible. The most recent biographer of Malthus, for example, states categorically, "Contraceptive practices could not become general until the vulcanization of rubber made possible the mass production of a variety of hygienic appliances."[25] But the French evidence proves that this was not so. Basic preindustrial methods of contraception and abortion were responsible for the lowering of the French birth rate, and it would not be until the twentieth century that mechanical means would play a significant role. The demographic transition thus was not the result of a technological revolution; on the contrary, it was the success French couples already enjoyed in controlling family size by utilizing old practices which eventually led to a demand that produced new contraceptives that were even more effective. This was a complex process in which older methods of fertility control continued to be employed — by the highly motivated with renewed vigor — and were gradually supplemented but not supplanted, at least in the nineteenth century, by new techniques.[26] The methods included varieties of periodic continence, reliance on nongenital intercourse, coitus interruptus, and finally employment of mechanical means of contraception.

The most obvious form of continence was, of course, simple abstinence. Large numbers of couples presumably relied heavily on such self-control, but even so natural a method could be to a degree "institutionalized" by the husband and wife having separate beds, if not separate bedrooms. In the 1890s Dr. Auguste Lutaud asserted that because the poor always had to share the same bed it could not be expected that they would follow the injunctions of their social superiors to bridle their passions.[27] Lutaud implied that the middle and upper classes could more easily abstain; indeed were figures available on the number of single beds, today's conscientious quantitative historian would no doubt find some correlation with the fertility rate.

A second form of periodic continence was practiced while the woman was nursing. As noted earlier, we now know that the lactating woman does enjoy a margin of protection against a subsequent conception. But if this fact was only proven in the twentieth century, it was popularly believed in the eighteenth and nineteenth centuries. P.J. Boudier de Villermet in *L'Ami des femmes* (1758) lamented the fact that already many French women disdained both the bearing and nursing of children.

> One blushes at having many children, and one carefully keeps them far from oneself. Pernicious advice of a wantonness which completely violates the dictates of nature.[28]

In an attempt to woo women back to their duty, the author reminded them that if they in fact conscientiously nursed their offspring they would not be burdened with inordinately large families. Rousseau likewise pointed out that the murderously high infant mortality rate could be brought down if children were so cared for. In the nineteenth century a full-scale attempt to advance nursing and the accompanying spacing of births as an answer to the population problem was made by Charles Loudon in *Solution du problème de la population et la subsistence* (1842). French anti-Malthusians such as Leroux and Proudhon expressed their interest in such a natural method of fertility control. The importance of nursing as a form of family limitation was not simply due to the physiological consequences it had on the mother; its real impact came as a result of its being used to back up demands for continence by the male while the woman cared for her baby. Even in the twentieth century in the Saintonge, evidence was found of the taboo against intercourse during lactation in the maxim that a child who is late in teething does not want brothers and sisters.[29] In other words, until a first baby was weaned, one should refrain from producing a second.

Reliance upon the safe period in a woman's ovulation cycle was the third method of periodic continence. It was in the nineteenth century that the subject of ovulation was scientifically examined and an explanation of its relationship to menstruation advanced by medical men. This question will be returned to in a later chapter. Here it is only necessary to note that much earlier there existed popular beliefs linking the woman's cycle and conception. Laurent Joubert in *Erreurs populaires au fait de la médecine et régime de santé* (1578) devoted a chapter entitled "Against those who advise knowing the woman during her flowers, in order not to fail to impregnate her." Joubert attacked the practice both because it was against "les bonnes moeurs" and because "the woman is at that time unable to conceive, which is the principle end of copulation."[30] Two centuries later a Dr. Venel in *Essai sur la santé et sur l'éducation médicinale des filles destinées au mariage* (1776) asserted that the days immediately following the menses were the most appropriate for fruitful intercourse.[31] The days before and during the period were sterile. From such statements it appears that though a good deal of confusion still surrounded the relationship of ovulation and conception there was an avid interest in determining periods of both fecundity and barrenness. It is impossible to say if many couples did discover a reliable form of the rhythm method but it is apparent that such a discovery was pursued.

Turning from the various forms of periodic continence to reliance on types of nongenital intercourse — oral, anal, and manual sex — one is still dealing with infertile forms of sexual behavior for which no outside information is required. In Nicolas Venette's *La génération de l'homme ou tableau de l'amour conjugal* (1778) is the statement: "Nature has taught both sexes such positions as are allowable, and that contribute to generation; and experience has shown those that are forbidden and contrary to health."[32] Determining the extent of such practices is difficult, but it is nevertheless important to note that well into the twentieth century such maneuvers would be employed by those seeking sexual relief but ignorant or unsure of other contraceptive measures. In 1887 Dr. Dartigues, in comparing the birth control practices of the various sectors of French society, asserted, "In the working class, one satisfies oneself in general by Onanism or else loses oneself in the immodest ways of pederasty or maneuvers of all sorts . . . *in vaso indebito*."[33] In 1911 Dr. Auguste Forel commented that oral and anal sex continued to play an important role in conjugal intercourse.[34] Such "vices" were attributed by doctors in the main to working-class men; it was assumed that the middle-class man similarly disinclined to employ contraceptives would not subject his wife to such practices but have recourse to a prostitute.

Prostitution was acknowledged by many social observers as an institution that permitted in an indirect way a form of family planning. After a man had fathered the desired number of legitimate children, he could decide to lead a chaste conjugal life while seeking sexual satisfaction outside of the home. Dr. Henri Thulié declared that in the nineteenth century such a solution was not uncommon. "And as nature does not lose its rights, the male goes expending his life at all the crossroads of venereal love; it is still cheaper than domestic and virtuous pleasure."[35]

The last of the nonmechanical forms of birth control and by far the most important contraceptive technique up until World War I was withdrawal or coitus interruptus. At the turn of the century when Jacques Bertillon asked his medical colleagues for reports on their patients' contraceptive practices, ninety stated couples relied on coitus interruptus, five on douching, four on the condom, two on abortion, and one each on sponge and pessary.[36] It is not suggested here that these figures give an exact picture of the employment of birth control methods in the 1890s — no mention is made, for example, of the natural means of fertility control which have already been discussed — but they do give some idea of the importance of withdrawal as compared to mechanical methods. In the eighteenth century coitus interruptus was only mentioned when under attack, but by the nineteenth century commentators increasingly referred to the practice as a commonplace occurrence. The Englishman Francis Place declared in the 1820s that withdrawal was widely employed by French couples; his words were echoed in 1857 by Dr. Alexandre Mayer who declared that it had become "un usage presque général."[37] In 1863 the economist Joseph Garnier went so far as to provide a veiled defense of the act in a scholarly journal. In *La Terre*, written in 1870, Emile Zola presented the peasant girl asking her partner, as a matter of course, to promise to withdraw before ejaculation and so "cheat" nature. Dr. Dartigues in works of 1882 and 1887 asserted that such practices were harmful to women; physiologically, inasmuch as the male withdrew before the female was satisfied and morally, inasmuch as the woman now knew how to commit adultery without fear of detection. In 1891, however, Dr. Lutaud retorted that there was no evidence of coitus interruptus having any harmful side effects. In the last decades of the nineteenth century the practice was reported even in the most remote provinces. Dr. Boismoreau noted that in the countryside the boy was warned to "faire attention" and the sex act was terminated "extra muros."[38] Dr. Raymond Belbèze speaking of the peasants of Gascony and Quercy wrote:

> They currently employ Malthusian practices, they "cheat," as is said in the provinces: this word almost always signifies "coitus reservatus." One sometimes has — and much more often than is imagined (the Malthusian practices remaining rudimentary) — recourse to a well-known abortionist.[39]

The fact that coitus interruptus was well-known, even to villagers, was further testified to by the number of aphorisms based on agrarian analogies that referred to the practice: "Battre en grange et vanner à la porte." "Faire comme le meunier: décharge sa charette à la porte du moulin."[40] Describing the inhabitants of the villages around Toulouse in the 1870s, Lavigne morosely reported:

> The families exclusively preoccupied by means of becoming rich isolate themselves in a cold egoism, accepting as the basis of the improvement of their lot the systematic sterilization of marriage. Only one child is wanted. At the second one groans and laments; sadness and sorrow enter the home separating the wife and the husband; and the grandparents cry that when one has one child *it is necessary to leave the tools in the attic.*[41]

Coitus interruptus was the primary contraceptive technique responsible for the decline in the French birth rate, a fact that few demographers would now deny. But two points related to the practice have not received sufficient attention. The first is that although some historians have argued that past generations may have "forgotten" how to employ coitus interruptus it is quite obvious that it is a technique that each couple could devise for itself. Accordingly the argument that a knowledge of contraceptive methods has to percolate down the social hierarchy for the birth rate to be curbed is seriously undermined. The second is that although some historians have viewed the practice as primarily a male form of birth control, the quotations which we have cited reveal that the active participation of both spouses was involved; the woman was not passive and indeed frequently was the one to insist that her partner be "careful."[42]

The third method of fertility control was reliance upon some form of mechanical device — condom, sponge, pessary, or douche. The origins of the sheaths or condoms (made in the eighteenth century of animal intestine, in the late nineteenth of vulcanized rubber) remains a mystery.[43] The English attributed them to the French by calling them "French Letters"; the French returned the favor in referring to them as *redingotes anglaises*. The reluctance of each nation to claim the invention as its own was due to the fact that sheaths were first employed to protect the male against the venereal disease of prostitutes, not to protect the woman against pregnancy. Jean Astruc in his *Treatise of the Venereal Disease* (1737) stated:

> I am informed, that of late years the Debauchees in *England*, that set no bounds to their meretricious amours, make use of a little bag, made of a thin bladder, which they call a *condum* [sic]with this they arm the *penis*, that they may be preserved safe from the dangers of an engagement whose consequences are always doubtful. For they imagine, that being arm'd thus *cap-a-pé*, they may with great safety face the dangers of promiscuous venery.[44]

Even in the early nineteenth century when French doctors discussed the utility of the sheath, it was almost always in terms of its value in preventing disease. Thus doctors who refused to discuss contraception as immoral could talk about prophylactic devices as necessary evils. "It is a means that the final cause of all legal sexual intercourse repulses, that morality has had always to blame, but which certain circumstances and necessity sometimes makes tolerable, I mean, the condom."[45] And while domestic sexuality was always discussed by doctors in the gravest tones, they permitted themselves some levity when referring to an instrument of a casual liaison. "A poor umbrella," was the way in which Dr. Philippe Ricord described it, "that the storm can break or displace, and which, in all cases, guarantees one rather poorly from the rain, and does not prevent the feet from getting wet."[46] In *Nouveaux éléments d'hygiène* (1827) Charles Londe provided one of the medical profession's earliest defenses of the condom as a hygienic device. "The sale of condoms is not general enough; this precious preservative that religion can blame since it facilitates the pleasures that it reproves, cannot be praised highly enough by hygiene. It should be sold in all the small as in all the large cities: one should find it stocked by all pharmacists."[47] Londe reported that already by the 1820s the redingote anglaise could be purchased at the gallery of the Palais Royal at the *"marchands de taffetas ciré."* But the sheath's utility as a contraceptive was not ignored. In the *Dictionnaire des sciences médicales* (1820) F.V. Merat de Vaumartoise acknowledged its value in preventing infection and conception, although he still was thinking primarily of conceptions resulting from extramarital liaisons.

> Misfortunes of all sorts which are born of an unlucky fecundity and which are the despair of their victims and families, will be [with the use of the sheath] more frequently spared. Numberless evils the result of human weakness will be avoided; there will be fewer attempts at abortion, fewer infanticides, etc. How many advantages would result from the more frequent use of such a simple means.[48]

Even in the 1870s when Bertherand and Duchesne reported to the Société de médecine de Lyon on the manufacture of "condoms, capotes, rubans de sûreté, anticonceptions, gants d'amours," it was obvious that such devices were still associated in the public mind with venereal disease and prostitution.[49] Eight small firms employing Alsatian workers and using rubber imported from Manchester produced, in addition to balloons, enough devices to supply the French market. The sheaths were sold at the *marchands de tabac* or in bordellos for fifty centimes. Despite their immoral associations, their danger of breaking, and what Dr. Lutaud referred to as their unromantic nature, it was the cost of the sheaths that most restricted their usage. At the end of the 1880s Dr. Dartigues declared that they were widely employed by the rich but unknown to the poor.[50] New brands with such evocative names as "L'Explorateur," "Le Reveur," and "Le Délicieux" began to appear in the 1890s, but it would be well into the twentieth century before they replaced the easiest and most widespread form of birth control — coitus interruptus.

Although many men were introudced to the use of the condom by a prostitute, it was generally thought of as a male form of protection. Sponges, pessaries, and douches represented the female mechanical methods of contraception. Evidence of the employment of such devices can be traced back for several centuries. In a poem entitled *Les Satyrs* (1609) Mathurin Regnier described finding in a prostitute's room "la petite seringue, une esponge, une sonde."[51] Presumably reference was being made to similar contraceptives by Henri Estienne in 1566 when after describing the evils of abortions he concluded, "It is quite true that today many women no longer have need to come to this, because of the means of several preservatives which protect them from becoming pregnant.'[52] In the 1820s the English radical Richard Carlile asserted that French women made their own protective devices out of pieces of sponge, but only in the last decades of the century were similar commercial products available.[53] On the one hand, there were the *éponges de sûreté* and pessaries made of rubber produced by Meigs or Dumontpallier. Dr. Lutaud described them in 1891 as "the best preventive which can be placed in the hands of a woman" while admitting that there was often the problem of them not fitting properly.[54] On the other hand, there were the soluble pessaries usually formed of cocoa butter and quinine. These not only blocked the vagina but had a spermicidal effect. In pharmacies of the 1890s one could find the well-named "Antikid" brand of the German company of Frolich and Heinzé as well as those of W.J. Rendell of London and Sauter of Geneva. According to a 1910 investigation by Drs. Bardet and Dufau, the problem posed by the soluble pessary was that irritation could occur if douching did not follow its employment. Nevertheless, women liked them. "Now, from what we could learn, the greatest number appreciated these suppositories *because they allow them to avoid getting up in order to douche.*"[55] What this suggests is that women once employed douching along with some sort of pessary but moved on to simple use of the latter when their confidence in it grew.

Douching by itself gives only a limited margin of protection against conception — and only if employed both before and after intercourse — but the fact that the douche and the bidet enjoyed such popularity in France, the one country in the early nineteenth century with a declining birth rate, is suggestive. Foreigners were particularly struck — as indeed they continue to be — by the ubiquity of the bidet, a contraption which emerged sometime in the late seventeenth century. Even Arthur Young, the English agricultural reformer, found time to write in 1790: "A *bidet* in France is as universally in every apartment as a basin to wash your hands, which is a trait of personal cleanliness I wish more common in England."[56] Young exaggerated the number of bidets; the poor, because of the device's cost and the lack of running water in their homes, could not employ it. Young also ignored the employment of the bidet with douching solutions for contraceptive purposes. Marc Colombat de l'Isère did not. In

A Treatise on the Diseases and Special Hygiene of Females (1845) the latter warned:

> All these toilet vinegars, these essences, the astringent compositions and all these mysterious waters that perfumers have the talent to produce, under a variety of picturesque titles, should be proscribed by females who attach any importance to the conservation of their health.[57]

But women did not have to turn to retailers for douching products; a little vinegar or alum in water provided a suitable solution.

One tends to know more about the commercial types of contraceptives for the simple reason that they were produced, advertised, and purchased. Their cost and limited distribution would, however, restrict their use until the twentieth century to the upper and middle classes. The vast majority of French couples had to rely on simple coitus interruptus. Obviously it posed risks but so too did all the other methods. Robert Michels, the noted political scientist, was no doubt describing the fate of many who discovered the hazards of employing contraceptives when he wrote:

> One of my own friends has procreated every one of his five children — of whom three are still alive, and whom he would not lose for all the world — while using a different preventive measure. We have, then, here a wide field for discoveries and improvements.[58]

It was because of the lack of completely reliable contraceptive measures that so many French couples would have to fall back on abortion as a second line of defense against pregnancy, an issue to which we will return in a later chapter.

What was the effect of these new forms of fertility control on the birth rate? In most western countries the birth rate of 40 per thousand of the eighteen century only dropped after 1870 to stabilize at about 20 per thousand in the twentieth century. In France it was already down to 30.8 per thousand in 1821–1830 and 27.4 per thousand in 1841–1850. It was this "premature" decline which alarmed French observers. Some chose to believe that the number of births declined naturally as the country became overpopulated, but others pointed out that Britain, Germany, and Italy, which all had high birth rates, sent out important numbers of emigrants while France with its low rate welcomed immigrants. Some chose to attribute the decline in fertility to the reluctance of the French to marry, but others pointed out that France's marriage rate standing at 15.8 per thousand in 1912 was superior to that of Germany, England, and Italy.[59] The truth was that the French had simply decided to have small families and proved to be eminently successful in carrying out their desires. Viewed in isolation, the developments in French population growth appeared healthy enough. An average life expectancy of somewhere in the mid-thirties in the eighteenth century had been increased by about ten years in the nineteenth century. A total population of nineteen million in 1700 rose to twenty-one million in 1750, twenty-eight million in 1800, thirty-seven million in 1850, and thirty-nine million in 1900. The annual average rate of growth was 1 percent for the period 1700 – 1750, 0.6 percent for 1750 – 1800, 0.7 percent for 1800 – 1850, and 0.2 percent for 1850 – 1900. The annual number of births continued to rise until 1875. But relative to the rest of Europe, indeed relative to its previous rate of growth, France after 1850 was in decline. If France had maintained its eighteenth-century fertility level, it would have had a population in 1880 of eighty-eight million instead of thirty-eight million. In 1750 the nation made up 18 percent of Europe's population and had the largest population of any country in Europe; in the course of the nineteenth century it was overtaken by Russia, Germany, and Britain whose rates of growth were two and one-half times as great. Particularly frightening was the fact that France, a country in which 60 percent of families had two or less children from the 1870s on, grew only 12 percent between 1850 and 1900, while Germany advanced at a rate of 57 percent. In 1914 the sixty-six million Germans who faced thirty-nine million Frenchmen were not only superior in numbers but far more numerous in the younger age cohorts and so all the more prepared for war.[60]

These gross national figures were the ones most frequently bandied about in the demographic debate, but they cloaked important regional and class differentials.[61] The fertility decline was early and pronounced in the Paris basin, Normandy, and the western half of the country, but there remained islands of high fertility in Brittany and the Massif Central. These areas began to produce smaller families only after 1870; their tardiness suggests the importance of a whole range of variables — urbanization, industrialization, standard of living, literacy, access to communication, language, religiosity, land use, and inheritance customs. Almost all of these issues would be touched on by nineteenth-century commentators, but class differentials drew perhaps the greatest degree of attention. Not until the 1906 census were there firm data available on differences in family size according to class, but long before that observers were convinced of the fact that in general the number of children diminished as family wealth increased.[62] This in turn had an important impact on the way in which the debate on fertility was carried out. By 1850 most analysts conceded that the upper and middle classes could not be coerced into returning to the tradition of large families; could the working classes be prevented from following their lead? Almost every respectable public commentator voiced the hope that they could. The state for its part took practical steps to support such sentiments by, on the one hand, elaborating a variety of social assistance schemes in an effort to "buy" babies from the working classes and on the other, outlawing any attempt to inform them about means of contraception. It was natural enough that successive French governments would seek to assure themselves of a populous work force at home just as they sought populous allies abroad—such as Russia—as counters to Germany. More surprising was the fact that such policies should be accompanied by attacks on family limitation when any intelligent observer had to be aware of both the widespread desire to limit pregnancies and the availability of means to accomplish such ends.

PART TWO

The Conservatives

CHAPTER TWO

French Catholicism and the Nineteenth-Century Birth Control Debate

Why, despite its wide employment, was there such public hostility to birth control in nineteenth-century France? Who opposed the spread of contraceptive practices? To such questions most educated laymen would probably respond that opposition to the limitation of births was based on traditional Christian teachings and that the defenders of such opinions in France were obviously the Catholic clergy. To test the assumption that the Catholic church took the lead in expressing open hostility to birth control the attitudes of the clergy will be analyzed in this chapter; in chapter three the position of doctors — who one might expect to be less antagonistic — will be examined; and finally in chapter four the views of secular moralists will be discussed.

What stance was adopted by the French Catholic church in the nineteenth-century birth control debate? Given the clergy's clear denunciations of contraception in the twentieth century, it is easy to assume that their views were, if anything, even more negative in the nineteenth.[1] Evidence to support such an opinion is readily available. In the years immediately preceding the First World War, birth control propagandists castigated the church for having opposed every attempt to limit the burdens of childbearing; the clergy, for their part, gloried in their self-appointed role of traditional defenders of the large family. But the real story is not quite so simple. In the first place, although the nineteenth-century lay and clerical molders of Catholic thought never defended *artificial means* of fertility control they did extend and modify their definitions of *natural means* of restriction. Second, and more important, the avowed interests of the church that legitimated its intrusion into the discussion of fertility shifted. In the first half of the century the church followed a relatively liberal line because it took as its chief concern, not family size, but the moral consequences of the actions of individual couples; it was only in the latter half of the century and especially after 1870 when the French church was swept along by the nationalist fears of depopulation that the now familiar conservative tack was adopted, manifesting itself in the preaching of the necessity of large families. To understand fully French Catholic views on birth control in the nineteenth century these two contradictory currents of thought have to be disentangled.

Catholic opposition to contraception was based on the traditional Christian teaching that the only lawful purpose of intercourse was reproduction. God had given the command to "Increase and multiply." But over time Christians also accepted that the intercourse of married couples could serve subsidiary, legitimate purposes in preventing adultery, maintaining health, and even in providing pleasure; all helped to mitigate concupiscence. From the Reformation on, however, Catholic and Protestant teachings slowly drifted apart. Both churches continued to accept the doctrine that it was God's wish that man multiply, but in the Catholic case the obligation of the laity was theoretically more pronounced because the priest performed the complementary act of celibacy. It was the continuance of celibacy that required the Catholic priests to broach sexual issues that Protestant pastors could discreetly avoid. It has been suggested that because conjugal life was a private affair in Protestant areas such as the Vaud, parts of Switzerland, and Hungary, restriction of family size from the eighteenth century on was largely a response to economic pressures.[2] Part of the Calvinist theological revolution had been the provision of a new picture of marriage in which the bearing of children was no longer the primary goal but a secondary consequence of marital harmony. In short pleasure and reproduction began to be distinguished as separate spheres. In Catholic France the bearing of children continued to be viewed as the primary purpose of marriage and this obliged the priest — unlike his Protestant counterpart — to question the actions of infertile couples. In Protestant Europe, although the artificial restriction of family size was considered in some general sense to be a moral issue, the extent to which the churches managed during the nineteenth century to ignore the question was striking. Such a blind eye could not be turned to the problem in Catholic France.

The Catholic church was initially drawn into the fertility debate, not because of a concern for population growth, but because of its necessary interest in the moral actions of its parishioners. A seventeenth-century catechism contained the injunction,

> It is really necessary to teach the married that the blessing of marriage is
> not only to have children, but to have children who will serve and fear
> God, and who can one day replace the Fallen Angels.[3]

In short the church was not blind to the burdens imposed by unnecessarily large families and from the mid-eighteenth century on accepted abstinence as a legitimate method of fertility control. There were, of course, always those who would regard even a cessation of intercourse as a sign of lack of faith. Père Féline declared in 1782:

> Providence is charged with furnishing means of subsistence to the poor. It takes pleasure in blessing their families while those of the rich perish . . . It is necessary to give oneself up to Providence, to put one's confidence in It.[4]

The Abbé Jaubert took an equally hard line in asserting that it was primarily the wealthy who restricted family size,

> in order to have a rich heir who will pass on to posterity their name and their power. It is thus in order to perpetuate an unbridled luxury, that one is deaf to the cries of nature, and prefers not to multiply the number of children.

But despite his self-righteous tone Jaubert admitted that few could be expected to heed his call: "Coquettish mothers will regard us as a savage who is ignorant of the maxims of the century and does not know his manners. Bachelors will treat us as a misanthrope."[5] It was in fact true that even the church accepted marital continence as a natural, legitimate measure when taken to avoid misery.[6] Accordingly the church could feel both morally and scientifically correct when Malthus advanced much the same argument at the end of the eighteenth century in his writings on population. The English parson and economist, it will be recalled, was opposed to artificial means of fertility control and declared that only by late marriage and abstinence could the poor hope to improve their conditions. Some French Catholic social commentators like Charles de Coux and J.P. de Villeneuve-Bargemont went so far as to assert that Malthusianism and Catholicism were complementary doctrines because only the true faith could provide the "moral restraint" for which Malthus called.[7] Similarly the leading Catholic economists such as Joseph Garnier and Frédéric Passy who defended Malthus's population theories did not proceed, as did the neo-Malthusians, to defend birth control.

Abstinence was accepted by the church as a legitimate method of restricting family size; artificial methods — the most widely employed being coitus interruptus or "onanism" — were not. Père Féline, previously cited, faithfully conveyed the church's teachings when he categorically condemned in *Catéchism des gens mariés* (1782) all obstacles to generation. These he listed as sexual excesses, premature ejaculation, noncoital positions, and onanism. The employment of such practices he attributed to women's distaste for childbearing and to

> the too great obliging compliance of husbands for their wives; they make themselves too sensitive to the complaints that wives make of all that it

costs them to bring children into the world. They [the husbands] treat
kindly their wives' excessive delicacy, they seek to spare them this pain
without, however, renouncing the right they believe they have of
satisfying themselves.[8]

Such spouses, Féline declared, had to be informed of their moral duty to
reproduce.

Féline's dogmatic injunctions could not be followed up. The
Revolution and the wars of the republic and empire crippled the French
church. When it slowly began to reassert itself as a leader in moral matters
in the nineteenth century, its tone was muted.[9] The moral theology that
was presented in the works of Jean-Baptiste Bouvier, bishop of Le Mans,
and Thomas Gousset, bishop of Rheims, tended to follow on questions of
marriage the lenient, non-Jansenist views of the Italian theologian St.
Alphonsus Ligouri (1697–1787).[10] Nevertheless, it was the French clergy
who took the lead in asking the Vatican to declare the guidelines to follow
on the issue of contraception. The early decades of the nineteenth century
were the years in which birth control was first openly defended in Britain
and America, but it was not Anglo-Saxon, neo-Malthusian ideas but
French practices to which the clergy was responding. The answers
provided by Rome were slow in coming and rather vague because the
term *onanism* continued to be used to describe both masturbation and
coitus interruptus. For the church the latter practice posed two problems.
First, since congregations were overwhelmingly female, priests wanted to
know if the wife could be held responsible for what was assumed to be a
male act. In 1816, 1822, and 1823 the Penitentiary (the Vatican office
dealing with questions of penance) replied that the wife's passive
acquiescence was not necessarily a sin if a greater evil was thereby
avoided. In 1842 when Bouvier sought further clarification, he was
directed back to the 1822 judgment. The Holy Office of the Inquisition did
determine in 1853 that the wife's passive acceptance of a husband's use of
a condom was a sin.[11] The second problem posed for the church by
contraceptive practices was that a too heavy-handed condemnation of
obviously widely employed methods could split a body of believers in the
very process of reuniting after years of revolutionary turmoil. The church's
refusal to declare categorically the wife's involvement in coitus interruptus
to be a sin reflected not so much its underestimation of women's interest in
controlling fertility as its prudent calculation that such a step would drive
from the confessionals important numbers of female parishioners. The
same caution led the church hierarchy to rein in zealous young priests
intent on closely interrogating the mothers of small families. Bouvier
recognized that many otherwise loyal parishioners restricted fertility,
believing in good faith in the moral innocuousness of the practice.[12] The

Penitentiary supported Bouvier's observations by declaring that the chaste and faithful were not to be offended by intrusive questionings. In short, the church accepted the view that "contraception could be practiced in innocence of its malice" — better that the married sin in ignorance than that they be forced to sin knowingly.[13]

The above line of reasoning, though accepted by the church hierarchy, appeared too equivocal to some. Accordingly, interest was expressed within the church when scientists reported at mid-century that in addition to abstinence, coitus interruptus, and employment of condoms there was a fourth natural method of limiting family size — reliance on the sterile period in woman's monthly cycle. A summation of popular Catholic attitudes on the acceptability of methods was presented in a text by Dr. Dufieux in 1854. Intercourse, he stated, was in itself degrading — he referred to "l'indignité de l'acte copulateur" — unless blessed by the church. All the more reason why the church could not bless acts "de l'onanisme conjugal" to which both rich and poor had recourse — the former to become richer, the latter to escape poverty.[14] Abstinence was a legitimate means of avoiding misery, but according to Dufieux, in the great majority of cases couples resorted even to this method to pursue wealth and pleasure. Onanism was of course worse because it represented a crime against God and nature; it symbolized man's futile striving for omnipotence and the triumph of destruction over production. The practice was unfortunately now so common in all classes that the traditionally large family had become a source of amusement to "all the ranks of a society accustomed to smile with pity at the conjugal crown with which God honors chaste spouses."[15] The practice of onanism was only the first step on the path to debauchery; the husband habituated to one vice, would soon demand others, the wife's refusal of which would drive him into the arms of prostitutes.

Dufieux showed no lack of imagination in picturing the potentially evil consequences of onanism, but at the same time he asserted that the desire of some couples to avoid additional pregnancies was understandable and legitimate. The church's main concern was morality, not population. Indeed, Dufieux estimated that on average only a sixth of all biologically possible children were born. It was neither crime nor continence that kept numbers at a reasonable level but the fact that God in His wisdom endowed women with a constitution that was only fecund at certain times of the month. The exact timing of ovulation was still something of a mystery, but Dufieux's clear implication was that here was a method of naturally controlling fertility. Dufieux provided an account of the scientist P. Cazeaux's work on ovulation to show how Providence in placing a sterile period in the female monthly cycle provided a legitimate way to avoid overly large families.

The scientific observation of the ovulation cycle took place in the nineteenth century, but the belief in its relationship to reproduction can be traced back over fifteen hundred years. Interestingly enough, St. Augustine, the first Christian thinker in the West to provide a full theological account of the problems posed by contraception, condemned the reliance on the sterile period as practiced by the Manichees.

> Is it not you who used to warn us to watch as much as we could the time after purification of the menses when a woman is likely to conceive, and at that time to refrain from intercourse, lest a soul be implicated in the flesh? From this it follows that you consider marriage is not to procreate children but to satiate lust.[16]

A similar attack on what can be called the "rhythm method" appeared half-hidden in the clotted prose of an anonymous tract of 1859, which castigated Jules Michelet for interesting himself, not in love, but in female physiology.

> But if, under the pretext of hygiene, you wish, o young man, to instil in your wife a *modern mind, believe* yourself to be the *sole possessor* of the truth in thinking only of *sensualism* and *animalism*, if you *believe* that your chaste and pure wife is only *gloomy* when she *believes* in God and in his *holy law*, that she has only learnt that which it is *necessary to forget*, her generosity, her *virgin nature* will be of no use except to lose both your child and the future, because the authority of your science, your knowledge, will only be the science, the knowledge of madness, of delirium, of misfortune.[17]

This outburst, if it was in fact an attack on the rhythm method, was not typical of mid-century Catholic reactions. Even Augustine's hostility was forgotten or overlooked while the writings of scientists such as Pouchet, Raciborski, and Cazeaux who dealt with ovulation were read with interest by Catholics worried by the spread of other methods of contraception. In 1853 Antoine de Salinis, bishop of Amiens, reported that some married persons, "relying on the opinion of skilled doctors," were persuaded that there were times of the month when conception could not take place. Asked its opinion of such practices, the Penitentiary replied guardedly that "those about whom you ask are not to be disturbed provided that they do nothing by which conception is prevented."[18] In 1867 when Dr. Avard again queried Cardinal Gousset as to the legitimacy of the rhythm method, another confusingly noncommittal answer was provided. Gustave Le Bon, the Catholic social commentator, was confident enough, however, of the implied meaning of Gousset's response to declare in *Physiologie de la génération de l'homme* (1868) that the church approved of the method.[19]

Finally in 1873 Auguste-Joseph Lecomte, a Louvain theologian, provided a full defense of the practice in *L'ovulation spontanée de l'espèce humaine dans ses rapports avec la théologie morale.* Lecomte's argument was based on the premise that reliance on the woman's sterile period was a "natural" method of contraception inasmuch as it was only a refined form of periodic abstinence.[20] The authorities' response was still somewhat ambiguous, but it was left to be understood that if the practice was a sin it was at least a lesser sin than that committed by users of contraceptives. Confessors thus had an alternative means to offer couples by which to prevent conjugal onanism, restore peace to families, and stop the commission of a "faute grave." Such was in essence the conclusion of the Penitentiary in 1880. The rhythm method under discussion was, of course, based on what would later prove to be faulty calculations, and the practical importance of its employment was probably limited.[21] On the theoretical level, however, the discussion was of great significance. It revealed that the church hierarchy was not indifferent to the desires of thousands of faithful Catholics to limit family size. For most of the century the bishops had shown a good deal of tact and moderation in dealing with an especially sensitive issue.

The reluctance of the church to delve too deeply into the marital affairs of its parishioners and the interest it showed in the rhythm method were both manifestations of a desire on the part of the hierarchy to accommodate in some way the obvious intent of French couples to avoid overly large families. There was within the church, however, also an anti-Malthusian current of thought which declared the technical details of *how* births might be avoided to be of scant importance; the real threat of a decline of faith in God's bounty was posed by the very idea that births *should* be avoided. This more conservative line of thought would eventually predominate, not so much because of any new hostility to contraception per se but because of a growing fear of anti-Christian modernism — materialism, socialism, feminism — of which birth control seemed only a symptom. Two aspects of this current of anticontraceptive Catholic thought are worthy of note. The first is that the most intransigent hostility to fertility control was at the start manifested by laymen and the lesser clergy; only very late in the day did the bishops embrace the new doctrine. The second point, which follows from the first, is that the dangers posed by birth control were increasingly declared to be more of a social than a moral nature. Accordingly, the church found that by the end of the century it was not alone in attacking such practices; it had been joined by a host of conservative and nationalist critics. Indeed, by the outbreak of World War I Catholic concerns were in large part submerged in and subsumed by the nationalist campaign against depopulation.

Central to the Catholic conservative view of fertility control was the argument that Malthus's doctrine, far from being a moral message, carried seeds of subversion. As early as 1840 the Catholic social commentator H.A. Frégier asserted that those who advised workers that their security rested not on their faith in God but on their ability to limit family size were endangering society. Abstinence was not possible in the slums and Frégier warned that the only consequences of attempts at birth control would be the desertion of families and the demoralization of labor. Sexual temperance would not be increased; greater immorality would be the more likely result.[22] A similar message was carried in the Abbé Corbière's article "Le Malthusianisme" which appeared in *L'Ami de la religion* in 1858. Castigating the French disciples of Malthus such as Joseph Garnier, Corbière maintained that Malthus's bleak portrayal of man's life on earth led to a loss of faith in Providence that could well be turned to the purposes of socialist criticism. Class antagonisms were severe enough in France; to expose the workers to Malthus's pessimistic prognostications could only make matters worse.[23]

Women were as likely as workers, so asserted other Catholic observers, to be led astray by the discussion of fertility control. As noted earlier, Père Féline warned in the late eighteenth century that women endangered the family by seeking to free themselves from the burden of childbearing. This argument was returned to at mid-century. France, it was declared, had become a Catholic nation because of the activities of a woman — Clothilde who cajoled Clovis into conversion — and if French men were to be returned to the faith, it would have to be at the instigation of their wives and mothers. But the faith of women seemed to be wavering. In their ignorance they were threatening the family structure, which was the basis of society. What was required was a suitable education for the woman to prepare her for the grave duties of motherhood and woo her away from the temptations of sending her child out to nurse and of relying on birth control to limit the number of her children.[24] The canon L.E. Bautain attributed the supposed enervation of middle-class women to more than their mindless seeking of pleasure:

> Behind all this there is still something even more deplorable, even more immoral, and something that we hardly dare indicate; one subordinates the goal of nature to its means, and one even turns the means against the end, in sacrificing the duties of maternity to the pleasures which assure it.[25]

The failure of confessors to tackle the issue was noted by Marie-Jean Guyau who claimed that the Jesuits closed their eyes to the existence of small families. Upper-class women were particularly zealous in limiting births.

> The ambition of upper-class women being too often, as one knows, to copy the manners of the *demi-monde*, it followed that they imitated them in this way as in all others, and that they sought to establish between marriage and prostitution this new similarity — infertility.[26]

If this were not bad enough, Guyau claimed that now even working-class women were employing the same practices.

> From the moment that woman thinks in place of allowing herself to be guided by faith, she cannot fail to sense the very great disproportion which exists for her between the joys of love and the sufferings of maternity. It is necessary that a new idea intervene, that of duty, and not only a religious obligation, at which the husband can sneer, but a moral obligation.[27]

The question Guyau posed was whether the church could adequately champion the population interests of France.

Conservative Catholics held that the discussion of birth control by workers was but one aspect of socialism while the interest shown in it by women was but one aspect of feminism. Ironically enough, however, the church found itself having to respond to the charge that its own institutions of celibacy and the confessional were themselves causes of depopulation. This provided yet a third reason why from the mid-century on Catholic writers felt obliged to speak out more forcefully against fertility control. In the eighteenth century the philosophes were quick to condemn ecclesiastical celibacy as one of the causes of France's presumed population decline. Montesquieu, Voltaire, Rousseau, and Mercier assailed celibacy as "unnatural" and such attacks were carried on into the nineteenth century by anticlericals like P.J. de Béranger and P.L. Courier, the latter for example, accusing priests of suffering from *"érotomanie."*[28] These charges were answered by Joseph de Maistre and Louis de Bonald, but neither writer declared that it was the church's intent to promote large families.[29] Such a note was only sounded from the mid-century on when real fears began to be expressed concerning France's slow population growth. Thus in 1854 Dr. Dufieux argued that the celibacy of priests strengthened Christianity, which in turn promoted fruitful marriages. In response the anticlerical Dr. Paul Diday replied that if such was the case why was it that the Protestant countries had a faster growth rate? Answering his own question he stated that it was because the Protestant clergy in marrying raised the marital state in public esteem; the Catholic clergy in defending celibacy could only undermine the public's view of fertility.[30] When the depopulation issue was rekindled at the end of the century, celibacy was again debated; Arsène Dumont and Roger Debury argued that Catholicism was a force for depopulation, with Camille Ract and D.M. Couturier violently denying it.[31] The century-long debate is of interest because whereas celibacy was presented by Catholic writers in the first decades as having primarily a moral importance, by the last decades it was also portrayed as having a practical impact on population growth. That it was difficult to demonstrate the positive effects of celibacy would be one more reason why Catholic writers, anxious to prove their concern for France's population growth, would come down even harder against contraception.

For the nationalists the defeat of the French by the Prussians in 1870 turned the mild concern for France's diminishing birth rate into agonizing soul-searching. The Catholic church was swept up in the populationist campaign because it appeared that here was an issue that could be used to win back the nation to its original faith. At a Bastille Day speech in 1872 Gaspar Mermillod, a Swiss cardinal, informed his French audience, "You have rejected God, and God has struck you. You have, by hideous calculation, made tombs instead of filling cradles with children; therefore you have wanted children."[32] When further requests for advice on how to deal with contraceptive acts were sent off to Rome by the French clergy after 1870, they were thus colored by nationalist preoccupations. They elicited a harsher response. In replying to pastoral queries of 1876 and 1886, the Penitentiary slowly swung round to the new view that the purported "good faith" in which believers employed contraceptive practices could no longer be used as a legitimate defense of their actions. If the naive were confused as to the immorality of fertility control, public interest now required that their good faith be questioned. In the first half of the century the church regarded the birth control issue as primarily a marital problem that had to be dealt with carefully and cautiously; by the latter half of the century the church began to view the question as a social problem that had to be met with strong measures. The clergy, on the one hand, aroused by the sheer increase in the incidence of contraceptive practice and its association with socialist, feminist, and anticlerical doctrines, and on the other sustained by the belief now held even by nationalist nonbelievers that France's declining fertility was the nation's major weakness, were emboldened to speak out more forcefully against such vices.

The lower clergy took the lead in adopting the more intransigent attitude toward contraception. The hierarchy, either because of its distaste for the subject or because of its prudent concern to await Vatican instruction, long remained silent. An example of the sort of vigorous attempts made by the more humble priests to challenge the "good faith" in which believers practiced contraception was the Abbé Hoppenot's *Petit catéchisme du mariage* (1908). In it the question of whether Malthus's belief in the danger of overpopulation was well-founded received the answer:

> The crisis to fear, at the moment, does not stem from the surplus of population, but from the surplus of production. The markets are swamped with products. There are not enough consumers for the provisions. The land, needing men, calls for settlers.
>
> Q. — Are there in our time heirs of Malthus's doctrine?
> A. — Yes, they are the neo-Malthusians. More treacherous and more dangerous than their master, they are currently spreading throughout all France their shameful doctrines. They go saying over and over again to the population that the deliberate limitation of children is a guarantee of domestic happiness and well-being. In order to introduce their criminal theories into public behavior, they have recourse to tracts, to lectures with slides. There they cynically teach the means of limiting the fecundity of mothers. Scientific means they say; in reality, barbaric and murderous means.
>
> Q. — What is the result of this antihuman propaganda?
> A. — The increasing decline of the population of France. The rich sensualists have welcomed with enthusiasm this theory which so well favors their egoism and vanity. One heir (two at the most) in order to carry on their name and their undivided fortune, that is what perfectly matches their low aspirations; that is what is sufficient for their shrunken, withered heart; that is what allows them, tirelessly and effortlessly to enjoy good cheer, to live in style, to live here below without concern or care, an easy and satisfied life.[33]

Such attacks on birth control differed remarkably from those of earlier times. Whereas in the past these practices were judged simply as a sign of a lack of faith or an excess of sensualism, now the clergy in addition attributed them to the machinations of neo-Malthusians, Masons, Jews, socialists, and feminists all bent on weakening France at home and crippling its colonialist expansion abroad.

In Belgium Cardinal Mercier gave the hierarchy's sanction to the anticontraception campaign in his 1909 tract *Les Devoirs de la vie conjugale*. French bishops on occasion spoke out as individuals on the issue but never before the war as a collectivity. Étienne Lamy of the Académie française attributed their timidity to the continued fear that too sharp a pronouncement would spark a revolt of the faithful.[34] Alfred Krug complained in 1918 that so many respectable people employed contraceptives that "the priest has to treat them with an indulgence unheard of in the good old days."[35] It required in fact the enormous bloodletting of four years of war to drive the French bishops into finally making a formal condemnation of all forms of contraception. In 1919 they declared:

> The principal end of marriage is the procreation of children; for this, God honors the spouses by associating them in his creative power and paternity. It is to sin seriously against nature and against the will of God to frustrate marriage of its end by an egotistic or sensual calculation. The theories and practices which teach or encourage the restrictions of birth are as disastrous as they are criminal. The war has forcefully impressed upon us the danger to which they expose our country. Let the lesson not be lost. It is necessary to fill the spaces made by death, if we want France to belong to Frenchmen and to be strong enough to defend herself and prosper.[36]

Birth control was declared by the bishops to be (to paraphrase Talleyrand) more than a sin; it was an unpatriotic blunder. What France required, asserted the bishop of Versailles, were not just virtuous families but "des familles nombreuses."[37]

It was by this circuitous route, marked by shifting preoccupations, that the French Catholic church arrived at its twentieth-century position on birth control, a position more than supported by Pius XI's *Casti connubi* of 1930.

Was the church successful in following a line which would win the favor of the faithful? It is a difficult point to determine. In the first half of the century the départements of greatest religious piety correlated to those of highest natality, but after 1870 the fertility of even the most devout regions of Brittany, the North-West, and the South followed the national decline. It has been held that Catholicism, by instilling stoicism, generosity, and faith in the afterlife, retarded the drop in the birth rate, but once Christian beliefs began to be eroded fertility fell. The argument can, of course, be reversed; the attempts to control procreation could have been a major cause of a loss of religious faith. But both of these scenarios share the common assumption that the teachings of the church remained static while the actions and ideas of its flock evolved. What this chapter has attempted to demonstrate is that in fact the church's teachings were also altered in important ways. Its lenient view of fertility control was gradually replaced by intransigent hostility; what once had been designated a minor fault was now portrayed as a serious sin. Why had this shift occurred? It is difficult not to conclude that the increasing Catholic rigidity was prompted as much by political and social preoccupations as by moral concerns. By attacking birth control, the clergy saw itself doing battle with the forces of modernism dedicated to the destruction of the church; by parading its fears for France's population growth, it saw a means of retaining the support of nationalists and conservatives. Given this evolution in Catholic teachings, it is possible to suggest that if the falling away of church attendance was due to unhappiness with the teachings of the clergy on fertility, the decline was as much due to the new aspirations of the church as to those of its parishioners.

CHAPTER THREE

Medical Attitudes
Toward Sexual Behavior

It is generally recognized that contraception was practiced on a wider scale in France in the late eighteenth and early nineteenth centuries than in any other part of western Europe. It has been suggested that the decline of the church as a moral force and the dissemination of rationalistic thought provided a context in which contraception was at least thinkable. If this was in fact the case, the question is posed: why did no respectable French writer defend birth control publicly until Paul Robin published *La Question sexuelle* in 1878? In England the practice was championed as early as the 1820s and 1830s by Francis Place, Richard Carlile, Robert Dale Owen, and Charles Knowlton. In France, on the other hand, the champions of birth control were silent while its denigrators were extremely vocal. Where did the opposition to the practice come from in France? Those writers who have dealt with the question have focused primarily on the hostility of the Catholic church. What has not been given sufficient attention was the widespread secular opposition to population planning. Indeed the tendency to view the debate over birth control as a simple question of Christian morality versus individual desires has led scholars to ignore many of the more interesting social and cultural problems posed by the diffusion of contraception. Perhaps the most striking issue was that presented by the medical profession's response. Doctors generally accepted the demographic concerns of the populationists but were, not surprisingly, primarily concerned with the specific practices employed to limit family size. In this chapter the question of the doctor's relationship to the middle-class family up to the 1870s will be first sketched out, followed by an examination of the medical profession's views on contraception.

Medical literature provides one of the richest and, as yet, least tapped sources of information on the moral attitudes of nineteenth-century France. For the student of the history of the family, this literature is of special interest; it documents the process by which the medical profession, in its attempt to win respectability, sustained and strengthened the old myths of female inferiority. Though not discounting the significance of scientific and social forces, one purpose of this chapter is to examine the too often underestimated role played by prescriptive medical works in the growth of the Frenchman's "faith" in medicine.

In the first half of the nineteenth century the French doctor's record of triumphing over disease was not in itself sufficient to establish the credibility of medical science. Able to offer his patients few tangible benefits, he could only make himself an indispensable fixture of bourgeois society by becoming, in addition to its medical consultant, its moral counselor and confessor. Whether or not one went to a doctor was therefore as much a question of one's mental state as of one's financial ability.

In what follows I will use medical publications to show that it was general medical opinion that the crucial factor in winning the confidence of the bourgeois *père de famille* lay in convincing him that doctors could provide the advice necessary to assure the moral health of the household. To attract the attention of men impatient with the spiritually inspired moral injunctions of the clergy, they elaborated a morality of moderation based on utility. To allay the fears of the patriarch, resentful of the intrusion of any outsider in his private affairs, they declared that their discreet ministrations could ensure the order and tranquillity of the family better than any priestly injunctions. To win the confidence of the husband and father, they demonstrated that in addition to establishing scientifically the inferiority of women and the legitimacy of traditional sex roles, medicine promised to increase the sexual prerogatives of the male.

When nineteenth-century observers declared "the doctor is replacing the priest," they were always referring to the new role assumed by medicine on that terrain previously dominated by the dictates of religion — the area of sex and the family. The following statement by Dr. François Foy (1793–1867), chief pharmacist at the St. Louis Hospital in Paris, was typical of the frequent, fervent, unabashed claims of preeminence made by the medical profession in questions relating to the family and marriage.

> In fact, who will state the age, the physical and moral development, the temperament, the constitution, all the conditions in a word, indispensable to the accomplishment of the marriage, to the maintenance of it, without health being troubled by it, life diminished, morality offended? The doctor. Who will discover hereditary or other diseases, the vices of constitution capable of rendering the marriage impossible or not? Again, the doctor. Who will bring to a family divided by a disease acquired or given, by a suspected pregnancy, by an invincible repulsion, etc., the calm and happiness which previously reigned so completely and which doubt, jealousy, ignorance, have alone troubled? Still the doctor.[1]

Jean Cruveilhier, professor of pathological anatomy at the Faculty of Medicine in Paris, impressed upon his students in similar words the heavy responsibilities of the ministry they were about to undertake.

> The doctor is the most intimate confidant of families; before him all the
> veils of private life fall; it is to him that one reveals the sorrow of the soul
> so frequently a source of bodily ills, and on which he knows to apply a
> consoling balm. . . . How many times does the doctor prevent the awful
> crime which results in death to hide the fault that results in life! . . . Every
> day the doctor, by his wise counsels, reconciles divided families,
> prevents scandalous ruptures, helps with his credit, with his
> interventions, and even with his purse, his clients in misfortune; because,
> gentlemen, our patients become our friends, friends all the more dear
> the more unfortunate they are.[2]

The advice that the patient received from his doctor for the
maintenance of the moral health and happiness of his family was in all
likelihood not markedly different from that which the church had provided
— "moderation in all things." The only difference was that by presenting it
as a natural law rather than as a religious injunction the doctor had made it
acceptable to the enlightened.

The interest the French physician took in the sexual activities of his
patients was not unwarranted. His ability to penetrate into the most
intimate areas of personal behavior was of immense symbolic significance.
It was a dramatic demonstration of the confidence in which he was held by
the patient. Such confidence was not easily won. The medical literature of
the early decades of the nineteenth century is of particular interest in that it
makes it clear that doctors were convinced that their success, like that of
the priests, in gaining entrée to the French family hinged on bringing first
the woman, and then through her the child and the husband, under their
sway.[3] Doctors and laymen assumed that women, having frailer
constitutions and condemned to the illnesses associated with childbirth,
would provide the basis for the doctor's practice.

Medical science was thus used to substantiate rather than to challenge
old sexual stereotypes. The church had always presented the woman as a
morally weaker creature; the medical profession was now providing
evidence that she was not only physically inferior to man, but also
congenitally defective. She was found to be a small, weak, frail being. Her
bones and muscles were underdeveloped. Her nerves were oversensitive
and her brain undersized. Her head, with its dominant "attractive
faculties" was, according to the phrenologists, ill formed. Her nature,
declared the psychologists, was lymphatic and childish. All these failings
were, however, only secondary manifestations; the source of all woman's
ills was her procreative function. Man was occasionally influenced by his
sexual needs; woman was continually inconvenienced.[4] She was a
permanent invalid.

The happy moments of women are so rare and so short that one must leave them all their illusions in this regard, and it would be cruel to tarnish them by the image of pain. . . . she seems destined to pain; thus sufferings to be formed, sufferings every month, sufferings to become a woman, sufferings to become a mother, sufferings when she can no longer be one, sufferings, always and often peril.[5]

This lurid picture of the unclean, unhealthy, unhappy female seized the imaginations of contemporaries. Michelet described her in the chapter of *L'Amour* entitled "La femme est une malade" as humiliated by nature and tyrannized by her physical needs.[6] In the words of Alfred de Vigny she was "la femme, enfant malade et douze fois impure!"[7]

In portraying a woman's health in such an alarming light, doctors were reflecting the traditional belief in female inferiority, but they were also building up an argument to break the resistance of husbands opposed to their entry into the household. They did not hide the fact that their ambition, like that of the priests, was to interpose themselves between the husband and the wife.

We only advise them [women] to remedy promptly the dispositions of their sex and to hide them as much as possible from their husbands, not out of a lack of confidence which they owe them, but to leave them in ignorance of a multitude of little infirmities to which women are subjected. If I were a woman, said Dr. Tanchou, my husband would be the last one to know of my particular indispositions; only my doctor, other than my mother, would be informed of them. . . . Because of this, the first thing that she must do, after marriage, is to choose a doctor; it is the most important act of her life after the choice of a husband . . . he [the doctor] is the only man from whom she can hide nothing.[7]

The notion that the doctor by becoming the family counselor and, in particular, the confidant of the wife, was replacing the priest was expressed by numerous nineteenth-century commentators. The doctor offered his female patients consolations and encouragements which P.S. Thouvenel, physician and deputy during the July Monarchy, described as "la médecine morale."[8] Louis Huart declared, "The lady's doctor has in our days replaced the confessor; and he has gone further than the confessor, because he is the sovereign director of the soul and body of his client."[9] Michelet in reflecting upon the contemporary belief that the ambitions of the two professions necessarily overlapped, used the analogy with the doctor to describe the priest's control of the woman.

A great power, to be so necessary, always called, desired! to hold the two threads of hope and of terror, who draws the soul at will. Troubled, he calms her, and calm, he agitates her; she weakens little by little, and

the doctor is stronger, he senses it, he enjoys it. . . . There is for the one
to whom all natural enjoyment is forbidden, a somber happiness, a sickly
sensuality to exercise this power, to cause the ebb and flow, to desolate
in order to console, to wound, to cure, and wound again.[10]

The hostility of the bourgeois husband toward the confessor who used
the woman to penetrate into the innermost recesses of family life had
become, by the nineteenth century, a commonplace. As the doctor
increased his powers the question was raised whether he would prove
equally intrusive. The husband naturally feared the one man who could
legitimately take the greatest liberties with his wife. As early as 1708
Philippe Hecquet, the prolific medical writer, in *L'Indécence aux hommes
d'accoucher les femmes* had condemned the temerity of doctors and
declared that the death of the woman was preferable to cures humiliating
to nature and dangerous to virtue.[11] The idea that the woman and the
doctor had a symbiotic relationship, that they conspired to permit her to
avoid both the demands of nature and her husband, exercised the
imaginations of generations of male writers. Rousseau was convinced that
such intrigues were common. "The league of women and doctors has
appeared to me to be one of the strangest peculiarities of Paris. It is
through women that doctors acquire their reputations, and it is through
doctors that women have their way. One is quite rightly fearful of the sort
of skillfulness that a doctor needs in Paris in order to become
celebrated."[12] But what could the husband do? It was the woman who
chose the doctor, said Balzac, and the doctor, knowing instinctively that his
reputation could be made or broken by the wife, sought to please her. If
she wanted to avoid her conjugal duty, the physician could be relied upon
to find an excuse. "A doctor puts you back into the conjugal bed when it is
necessary, for the same reasons that he used to chase you out of it."[13]
Huart agreed; a doctor would not expose a woman who was using "une
bonne petite maladie nerveuse" to get her own way.[14] In the face of such
an alliance, grumbled Michelet, the husband was helpless. "If the doctor
orders it, the wife modestly lowers her head, and she resigns herself to it. If
it is the husband who prays and begs, she blushes, she becomes
indignant."[15]

Michelet's comments are especially revealing. No man was better
known in France than he for campaigning against the interferences of the
confessor in family life. He was, moreover, convinced of the benefits of
medical science. But now he was discovering, to his obvious
embarrassment, that the doctor was assuming the position from which the
priest had just been dislodged.

Our doctors are a class of extremely enlightened men, and, as far as I am
concerned, the first in France, without comparison. . . . But after all,

their rough masculine education in the school and the hospital, their severe surgical initiations, one of the glories of the country, all these qualities lead here to a grave problem. They extinguish in them the fine sensibility which alone can perceive, which can pierce, divine, the female mystery.[16]

This mystery was to remain the special province of the husband while any physical ills could be attended to by the women, Michelet suggested in a chapter of *La Femme* entitled "Puissance médical de la femme."[17] The austere utopian socialist Étienne Cabet supported a similar idea of medical segregation; male doctors for men and female for women.[18]

The suspicion about the doctor and female-patient relationship never completely disappeared but it became a minor theme because the medical profession provided abundant proof that its activities in no way menaced either the existing family structure or traditional sex roles. Doctors demonstrated that medical science could provide a host of modern utilitarian arguments to support customary social and sexual mores. The "medical morality" was to be as good as, if not better than, religious morality in inculcating acceptable social behavior. For example, the father whose sons were tempted by "vicious habits" was told by the doctor that in the modern age the injunctions of medicine were far more impressive than those of the church. "Assuredly, against an evil which depends on the will, the means of persuasion must be considered as the most efficacious. The fear of God, when it really and powerfully exists, suffices; but how rare it is! The fear of death and disease is often shown to be more coercive. . . . "[19] Dr. Philippe Ricord, the most famous investigator of venereal disease of the mid-nineteenth century, reported that his duties included assisting fathers to instill just such fears in their sons. "One knows that many fathers regard as a complement to moral education a visit to a venereal hospital, where they can say to a son who is about to make his entry into the world: 'Look and if you do not fear God, fear the pox,'"[20] The fear harbored by some husbands that through the activities of the doctor their wives might free themselves from their conjugal duties was also allayed. The doctor provided proof of female inferiority while showing how such weaknesses could be turned to the account of family stability; he defended the prerogatives of the male in the sex act; and most dramatic of all, he offered the husband the power of controlling procreation.

A French man who perused any of the popular medical texts produced in the first half of the nineteenth century would put down the volume with his belief in male superiority agreeably reinvigorated. The woman's procreative function, he was informed, doomed her to a semi-healthy existence that began at puberty and required the constant control and guidance of a male. The appearance of menstruation was a sign to the *père de famille* that his vigilance was necessary if his daughter's first sexual crisis was not to end in tragedy. He was warned that his daughter should be withdrawn from the *pensionnat* at once, for if she remained her companions would inevitably initiate her into the vice of masturbation.[21]

Many doctors believed that girls were as much given to "self-abuse" as were boys. J.J. Virey, a producer of many works of *littérature médico-philosophique*, claimed that the weaker sex was more devoted to the practice for the very reason that it was less closely watched.[22] Dr. Louis Seraine, who wrote a number of popular sex manuals, felt that the female habit, because of its prevalence, warranted a specific appellation, *clitorisme*.[23] The danger of female masturbation was that it could arouse an appetite for sensual pleasures that later legitimate intercourse would not satisfy. Similarly, doctors warned parents against permitting their daughters to read romantic novels or to view erotic plays; the drab reality of married life brought into sudden contrast with such dreams could result in hysteria.[24] The young girl was thus best served by the father who restricted her to a calm and sequestered life which occupied her mind and exhausted her body. The reading of history was useful, advised Lachaise, to enervate the more passionate natures.[25] The purpose behind these stratagems was not to destroy all female sexual feelings: it was to permit what society found tolerable, no more, no less. Accordingly, if a girl developed slowly, a father was advised on how he might best prepare her for the marriage market.

> A directly opposite plan should be adopted for girls who, though arrived at the nubile stage, are cold, apathetic, and indifferent; and, it is to such only that the culture of fine arts, the frequenting of balls, of theatres, of crowded assemblies, and even the reading of certain imaginative works and romances, will not be hurtful, and might even prove useful in exciting their sensibility, and thus inviting the menstrual exhalation.[26]

The very fact that the woman was subjected to a regular menstrual cycle was, declared doctors, proof that she lacked that complete freedom that was the true mark of humanity. The cycle was a subject of active investigation in the 1830s. The old idea, retained by Dr. Roussel, that it was not natural but caused by the intemperance and lasciviousness of women was losing official backing. Similarly the belief that the cycle was directly related to the phases of the moon, as were the tides, was less frequently expressed.[27] Nevertheless, the conviction that it was symptomatic of woman's proximity to the lower animals, that, like them, she was *in rut* during the menstrual period, was not shaken off. Even after F.A. Pouchet's pioneering work in the 1840s, the myth carried on. Though Pouchet understood the process of ovulation, his inference that a woman was most fertile for the week before and after her period was completely wrong.[28] The fact that his "schedule" was accepted and retained for the next fifty years, despite mounting contradictory evidence, must be attributed to the fact that his theory comfortably supported preconceived notions.

The woman's period was a repeated reminder of her physical incapacity. At such times she was no longer a simple *malade* but a *blessée*. For ten days before and after her *crise*, she, who was not as rational as man at the best of times, slipped even further back toward the irrational world of the child.[29] Here was a constant reminder of the husband's duty to retain firmly but gently the role, which could never be seriously assumed by his incapacitated mate, of head of the household.

Menstruation was not, however, to be viewed simply as a distasteful aspect of the female's biological life; doctors told their male readers that it was a natural function, the understanding of which could strengthen the family structure. Michelet understood the lesson that contemporary medical men were trying to teach the layman. Man had no divisions in his life; woman's life went on and on in a charmingly predictable cycle. "Everything is poetry in the woman, but especially this rhythmic life, harmonized in regular periods, as though stressed by nature." By observing and analyzing this rhythm, the physician had given the husband a more discreet but also more powerful means for controlling his spouse. Indeed, his knowledge of his wife's cycle permitted him to control her psychologically as well as physically. "The fertilization of the soul, as much as that of the body, requires that one do nothing except at the most favorable moments."[30]

According to the medical manuals, once a young woman had reached sexual maturity she had to marry, not simply because as a physically, economically, and intellectually weak creature she was likely to perish on her own, but also because her constitution could only support the demands placed upon it if her natural function, childbearing, were fulfilled. Underlying the reiterated statement that the female fully flowered only in marriage was the belief that the husband provided the wife with some of his excess "life force." Victor Hugo expressed this idea most clearly and crudely: "Man has received from Nature a key with which he rewinds his wife every twenty-four hours."[31] Doctors provided a medical explanation for this old notion by declaring that a woman needed a man's "vital fluid" if her own constitution were to be complete. "It is thus certain that the masculine sperm impregnates the organization of the woman, that it enlivens all its functions and heats them, that it gives more expansion and activity to her economy, that she feels better, at least if the excess of enjoyment does not enervate her."[32] Charles Lachaise and Charles Londe were somewhat more cautious in attributing specific chemical qualities to semen, but their interpretation of the therapeutic function of marriage was not radically different.[33] Marriage, by uniting a man, who had an excess of energy, with a woman, who had a deficit, was nature's way of reestablishing the equilibrium of human society.

Since woman received "energy" in marriage while man lost it, it was not surprising that doctors should prescribe marriage as a cure for a variety of female ills. Continence was declared to be the root cause of a host of female complaints, of which hysteria was only the most famous.[34] Lachaise wrote that he knew of cases in which a state of hysteria had been brought to an abrupt end by a simple offer of marriage. Dargir referred to it as "the best of all purgatives to chase away their [women's] bad moods."[35] Gustave Le Bon, writing in the 1860s, reported that doctors were still prescribing marriage and childbearing as cures for hysteria and uterine problems; the consequences were often disastrous.[36] Most doctors passed over such mishaps in silence while ridiculing the childless woman as *un non-sens dans la nature*.

Having provided an explanation of the physical and psychic workings of the female, doctors proceeded to advise the male on how he could, in responding to her demands, best preserve his health. Because they gave new life to the cherished notion that in the sexual act two distinct roles were played — man gave and woman took — they had also to deal with the old questions: Did women experience the same feelings as their mates, and if their satisfaction was any less, did this constitute a legitimate complaint? The doctors' answers were obviously designed to assuage the fears of the male who was having doubts about the competence of his performance. He was informed that he should ignore any female complaints of dissatisfaction; medical science had established that women were constitutionally unable to achieve the same pleasure as men. They did not expend as much energy in the act and it was thus natural, declared P.J.B. Buchez and U. Trélat, that they should not reap the same benefits. "Coition is infinitely less fatiguing for them than for man, they can more impudently repeat it . . . but their passions are not the less lively and their efforts are often the more damaging in that they are less satisfied; love is more frequently a cause of madness in women than in men."[37] Lachaise stated, "A rather large number [of women] only feebly experience pleasure, and none in the ordinary state feel toward the end of the act this kind of convulsive spasm which terminates it for us."[38]

Since women did not experience the same satisfaction and were not debilitated by the sexual act, a problem could arise if, in a futile effort to achieve fulfillment, they pushed their spouses to sexual excesses. The question of "excesses" revealed the medical profession's totally schizophrenic portrayal of female sexuality. In discussing the nature of such dangers, doctors developed the concept of what has been described as a "spermatic economy."[39] The man's capital, his vital fluid deposited in his *bourses*, had to be expended prudently. Excessive expenditures could result in moral and physical bankruptcy. "To diminish the sum of our pains as of our joys," wrote Virey, "is to slow the expenditures of life and economize our years."[40] In this bourgeois melodrama the woman appeared in the role of the profligate dependent who posed the danger of completely undermining her husband's corporeal economy by her extravagant demands. This fear of the woman was not new. The classic account of sexual mores written by Nicolas Venette in the seventeenth century, and frequently reprinted in the nineteenth, cautioned the husband against a wife's insatiable claims which could lead to a premature senility.[41] Dargir held up to abuse those wives who were guilty "of having wasted the health of their husbands and of having hastened their days by their extravagant appetites."[42] In the late eighteenth and early nineteenth centuries, doctors were providing medical justifications for such fears. A woman, stated Virey, gave man life by her cares but could kill him with her demands: "Either she prefers our conservation to her pleasures or she seeks her ecstasy at the price of our life."[43]

The picture that doctors presented of women's sexual appetites must have struck many readers as frightening. A man was held back from intemperance and debauchery, said the *normalien* V. Parisot, by his physical limitations; a woman only by her modesty.[44] Some doctors listed breast cancer, hysteria, and a variety of other ills as a consequence of *nymphomanie, fureur utérine*, and *érotomanie*, but others declared that women had nothing to fear from the sexual excesses of a monogamous relationship. And no matter what ills the wife suffered they could not approximate in gravity those of the husband. He was the one who lost the *fluid précieux* and accompanying nervous energy. He was the one who experienced sadness after coition: "it is a foretaste of destruction in past pleasure, but especially in that which transmits the gift of existence. Every animal after coition has given with effort a portion of his life, the rest is the part of death."[45] The image drawn by the doctor of the voracious female provided additional reasons why the husband had to control both himself and his spouse. When one recalls that the doctor advised the man to marry a girl several years younger than himself — Foy suggested ten to twelve years younger — it is easier to understand why the medical profession's counsels of moderation would be appreciated. The husband who restricted himself to the limitations laid down by the doctor could consider himself not weak but prudent; the husband who exceeded them could consider himself a prodigy.

Doctors advised men not only how to most effectively husband their physical energies, but also (as some physicians publicly advised by the 1840s) how to control the size of their families. What stood out in their discussion of the subject, however, was their hostility to the most widely employed form of contraception — coitus interruptus. To understand the physician's view it must be noted first that for the period in question there was no specific word for birth control. The term *onanism* was used to describe the "spilling of one's seed," be it by masturbation or by contraception. The book of Genesis states that Onan, though ordered by God to marry his dead brother's wife, "wasted his seed on the ground" each time he had relations with her, in consequence of which God killed Onan.[46] Biblical scholars long disputed whether Onan's punishment was due to his violation of leviratic marriage or to the specific means used. Nevertheless, Onan's name came to be associated with the sexual offense, not with the general problem of disobedience. Though Onan's act was clearly that of coitus interruptus, the term *onanism* was used primarily by doctors and priests to refer to masturbation; the withdrawal method of contraception was regarded as a subspecies of masturbation and was referred to as onanism or "conjugal onanism." The continued confusion over the proper use of the term throughout the nineteenth century indicated that birth control, though increasingly practiced, had not yet won sufficient public acknowledgment to warrant a distinct appellation.

The taboo against the spilling of seed existed in many cultures, Christian and otherwise, and consequently may have reflected a profound psychic fear present in most of humanity. In France in the latter half of the eighteenth century, however, this concern was for the first time justified on medical grounds. The man most responsible for viewing onanism in a "rational," non-metaphysical light was the Swiss physician Auguste Tissot, author of *L'Onanisme: ou dissertation physique sur les maladies produites par la masturbation.*[47] According to Tissot, the body was decaying every moment of our lives. Any exertion led to further decay, but sexual activity was the most costly. Man's seminal fluid was his most precious resource, animating every area of his constitution, and was in short supply. The loss of one ounce of sperm was equal to the loss of forty ounces of blood; equally damaging was the accompanying flight of nervous energy. Seminal fluid, because of its potent qualities, had to be expended but only in moderation. Legitimate, normal intercourse was in itself demanding, but a pleasure that could be indulged in repeatedly and that was not in some sense balanced by being part of a creative act was suicidal.[48] The physician's opposition to contraception and masturbation thus sprang from the same concern: neither act was limited by fear of offspring and so both would inevitably lead to sexual excesses.

Tissot listed a galaxy of diseases that ravaged the body weakened by self-abuse or by those sexual excesses that followed when there was no possibility of insemination. He related in horrific detail the case histories of youths who destroyed themselves through lack of self-control. Yet the remedies that the good doctor advanced were surprisingly mild: cold baths, clean living, healthy exercise. Indeed, an important factor in the popularity of the book was its stress on "self-help." The reader would now be able to recognize the telltale lassitude, loss of color, and sunken eyes, and take the appropriate action.

Tissot was not the first to indicate what he supposed were the weakening effects of semen losses; his importance and originality lay in providing for the first time modern medical "proof," independent of religious injunctions, to support the accepted belief that sexual excesses were bad. His application of natural, physical laws to explain the evils of onanism was an approach that clearly seized the imagination of his contemporaries. The author of the article "Manustupration" in the *Encyclopédie,* for example, faithfully followed Tissot in viewing masturbation as a simple medical problem.

> We consider it here only as doctors, as the cause of a multitude of very serious diseases, most often fatal, leaving to the theologians the care of deciding and making known the enormity of the crime. By considering it from this point of view, in presenting the awful picture of all the accidents it produces, we believe we can more effectively turn people away from it.[49]

After having listed the diseases that Tissot attributed to onanism, the author concurred that both conjugal and solitary vices had to be avoided at all cost.

> All these maladies are caused principally by the excessive evacuation of semen, coition and *manustupration* being regarded as almost equal; but observation makes it clear that the accidents that result from this illegitimate excretion are much graver and more prompt than those that follow the too often repeated pleasures of a natural relationship.[50]

For the next century every doctor who dealt with the problems of sexual intemperance was to base his case to a greater or lesser extent on Tissot's findings. Typical of such works were J.B. Pressavin, *Nouveau Traité des vapeurs* (1770); M. Contencin, *Consultation sur un onanisme* (1771); J.J. Doussin-Dubreuil, *Lettres sur les dangers de l'onanisme* (1813); Charles Malo, *Le nouveau Tissot* (1815); N.M. Buet, *Dissertation sur la masturbation et les moyens à y remédier* (1822); L. Rostan, *Cours élémentaire d'hygiène* (1822); F. Voisin, *Des Causes morales et physiques des maladies mentales* (1826); J.L. Alibert, *Physiologie des passions* (1826); Charles Londe, *Nouveaux élémens d'hygiène* (1827); and M. Audin-Rouvière, *L'Oracle de la santé ou l'art de se bien porter* (1829). These works added little if anything to Tissot's theory; that such tracts continued to be purchased was due in part to the fact that by the 1820s cheap illustrations were adding a new dimension to the terrible tales of sexual excess. An anonymous little book that came out in 1830 entitled *Livre sans titre* consisted of sixteen charming prints chronicling the physical decay of the onanist. In illustration seven the youth loses his teeth, by nine his hair falls out, in eleven he begins to vomit blood and by twelve breaks out in boils. Death claims the poor fellow at age seventeen, print sixteen.

The doctors' discussion of onanism in the nineteenth century was to differ in two important respects from that of the eighteenth. First, the physical harm associated with sexual intemperance was gradually downplayed, and greater stress was laid on the nervous disorders to which it could give rise. P.J. Forestier described the plight of a young man who "having married his wife in the summertime became maniacal as a result of the excessive intercourse he had with her."[51] Viewed as a cause rather than an effect, masturbation was to play a major role in the early psychological studies of Philippe Pinel and Jean Esquirol.[52] Second, whereas the eighteenth-century physician had tried to cure or prevent sexual excesses through correct diet and upbringing, his nineteenth-century counterpart placed greater stress on repressing the vice by the use of mechanical devices, medicaments, or surgery that culminated in the infamous cauterizations and clitoridectomies.[53]

The emphasis on the repression of onanism was exploited by quacks. Expanded publishing facilities were beginning to allow anyone to obtain a hearing, and new advertising schemes popularized miraculous medicaments. G. Jalade-Lafond was one of the first to plunge into this new medical market, offering to the public two antimasturbatory corsets in *Considérations sur la confection de corsets et de ceintures propres à s'opposer à la pernicieuse habitude de l'onanie* (1819). J.B. Téraube in *Traité de la chiromanie* (1826) reviewed a number of mechanical devices that could inhibit a child from touching himself, but he was most taken by Hippolyte Larrey's suggestion of injecting a substance into the uretha that would make contact with the genitalia painful.[54] Dr. Léop Deslandes provided similarly helpful information in *De l'onanisme et des autres abus vénériens* (1835).[55]

It is interesting to note that some of the quack literature was either written by English authors, or at least made a pretense of being directed at an English audience. This represented a part of the long tradition of Anglo-Saxons and Frenchmen attributing to each other esoteric sexual knowledge not possessed by their own countrymen. In 1836 Dr. Charles Albert published in Paris *The Doctor for Secret Disorders, or the Art of Curing Oneself*, containing lengthy testimonials from the satisfied imbibers of his "Sarsaparilla wine" and "Armenian Bole." Such charlatans played on the fear that masturbation and coitus interruptus were debilitating. In *De la virilité* J.L. Curtis printed what he claimed to ba a patient's letter, a rare first-person account of the withdrawal method of birth control. The anonymous letter writer declared that despite not having enough money to marry, he had been allowed to share his sweetheart's bed.

> I arranged it in such a manner that I could sleep with her two or three nights a week. The great respect in which I held both her and her family determined me to avoid the usual result of such a liaison, so that I always took care to withdraw before having completed the act.[56]

The technique had proved successful for over three years but then the price had to be paid for such excesses. The writer felt less vigorous and suffered from back pains and gonorrheal running. Fortunately a perusal of *De la virilité* enlightened the sufferer as to the cause of his complaint. Curtis's potion was sent for and within weeks full health was restored.

R. and L. Parry and Company, the creators of "Baume cordial de syriac," sought by a skillful combination of biblical texts and horrific illustrations that condemned and chronicled the life of the "self-polluter" to stampede the public into the purchase of their wares. Their main target was the masturbator, but the French male interested in controlling the size of his family could hardly rest easy after viewing prints of diseased visages and reading in *L'Ami discret:*

> The punishment incurred by those who disobey this order [to procreate] is the loss of the sentiment of pleasure, a punishment so harsh that few would care to face it. Nature has endowed us with a powerful disposition to carry out this duty: the human heart is revolted by those who denature this moral obligation imposed by the creator, who thus renounce the greatest portion of the joys of life. . . . Natural religion and our own reason should tell us that every action contrary to this object must offend God; that its consequences are terrible; that it destroys all conjugal affection, opposes natural inclinations and leads to the extinguishing of the hopes of posterity.[57]

Happily the fallen were not completely lost; they had a merciful savior and Parry's "Baume cordial de syriac."

To conclude this survey of the medical profession's view of onanism, one might turn to a more disinterested commentator, Dr. Claude-François Lallemand, author of the three-volume work, *Des Pertes séminales involuntaires.* Lallemand declared the mechanical prevention of masturbation useless and possibly dangerous;[58] he scoffed at the idea that simple coition was debilitating.[59] For the benefit of colleagues who as late as the 1840s still could not distinguish between masturbation and coitus interruptus he carefully delineated the two acts, saying of the latter:

> Every day, very scrupulous spouses do the same [as Onan] either in order not to increase the size of their family beyond their means, or because of the dangers that a pregnancy would pose their wives. There will be then here only the motives of Onan that one could disapprove. But the act in itself has nothing in common with masturbation.[60]

Had Lallemand thus freed himself from the common fear of sexual excesses? No. Though he did not consider any sexual act harmful per se, he was as adamant as his colleagues that semen losses constituted one of the greatest dangers to the nation's health. It was not the act but the number of times it was carried out that was important.[61]

In the passage cited above Lallemand mentions the husband's responsibility to his wife, which brings one to the question of the "antionanist" view of women. The literature attacking birth control is of particular interest in that it reveals a strong misogynist current running through both French medical and philosophical texts. The antionanists depicted the woman as a possible threat to her spouse and to society at large. The latter fear was based on the conviction that women, moved by licentious insouciance, were the ones most interested in birth control because it would permit them to avoid motherhood. Rousseau set this line of argument in declaring:

> Since the state of motherhood is onerous, a means is soon found of avoiding it altogether; the woman wished to do a useless task [i.e., have sex but avoid impregnation] in order to continually redo it, and to the harm of the species one turns the attraction given to multiply it. This practice added to the other causes of depopulation heralds the advancing state of Europe. The sciences, the arts, philosophy, and the mores that they engender will not take long in making it a desert.[62]

Rousseau's only consolation was that for the moment the practice was restricted to a "hundred large towns where women, living in licentiousness, bear few children."[63]

The belief that the woman was a threat to her spouse sprang from the old notion that each sexual act sapped the male's source of vital fluid. The *Nestor français* warned:

> Young men, no matter how you look at the seminal liquor you will recognize that of all our liquids it is the one most impregnated with

spirits, with life-giving elements not only necessary for the propagation of our species, but for the functioning of our intellectual faculties. It is an igneous fluid which, if too concentrated, burns us and rapidly devours us, but the wasting of which brutalizes and destroys us, morally, then physically; because it is its presence which develops our intelligence and gives energy and pleasure to our thoughts, as it gives vigor to our actions.[64]

An excessive loss, so the authors claimed, led to a drop in the body temperature, a slowing of the physical functions, madness, and finally death.

Women were necessarily inferior creatures, deprived as they were of vital fluid.[65] It followed that the female, being a passive partner in the sexual act, did not risk the same dangers but might drive her spouse on to sexual excesses. It was therefore necessary to instill in the woman modesty and obedience. J.A. Millot and A.J. Coffin-Rosny viewed any activity that broadened the woman's horizons as potentially harmful. They declared that intellectual stimulation was dangerous to females and undermined their health. The young girl was to be watched over by her parents and the church, exhausted by physical activities which would leave her indifferent to the investigation of her own body, and quickly married off "to put her morality in safety."[66] Marriage, according to the *Nestor français*, had as its object the propagation of the species, the maintenance of the social order, and last of all, personal happiness. To ensure all three the woman had as her task that of watching over her husband's precious supply of seminal fluid.

The marriage once consummated, a new career presents itself to the solicitude of the young wife; it is necessary that she have the courage of making her husband adopt a moderate usage of his pleasures which will ensure the longest duration of them and prevent the danger of an abortion or a premature birth.[67]

Thus, even at the moment of conception the woman was regarded as more an accessory than a participant in the creative act. There remained the fear, however, that even the best-trained woman would attempt to usurp the active role.

Calming the sexually aroused female was to be accomplished by both moral and medical means. In the latter category there is a small literature ranging from M.D.T. Bienville, *La Nymphomanie ou traité de la fureur utérine* (1786) to Dr. Rozier, *Des Habitudes secrètes ou de l'onanisme chez les femmes* (1825) to L.F.E. Bergeret, *Des Fraudes dans l'accomplissement des fonctions génératrices* (1868). In the latter work Dr.

Bergeret describes the practice of introducting into the vagina "des boulots de charpie imprégnées des substances calmantes, comme le laudinum ou le chloroforme." Bergeret's operation was not without its dangers. The good doctor sadly states that a medical friend eventually collapsed as a result of the emotional exhaustion brought on by having to repeat this operation at ever more frequent intervals on two hysterical girls.[68] The remedy advanced by Bergeret to cure every feminine complaint was pregnancy. The danger posed by the fraud of conjugal onanism was that the woman was raised to a high pitch of excitement, but then left unfulfilled, that is to say, not pregnant.

As long as conjugal onanism or coitus interruptus was the main method of birth control, doctors had nothing original to contribute to its discussion. Doctors did warn their patients against the sexual excesses that might occur if the woman were freed of the fear of childbearing; many attacked coitus interruptus as conjugal masturbation and attributed to it all the horrid consequences of self-abuse. Until the 1840s, however, the doctor had little to say about such habits that had not been said much earlier by the priest.

It was the appearance in the 1840s of several important studies of reproduction that permitted doctors to assume the role of specially qualified commentators in the Malthusian debate that so preoccupied nineteenth-century France. As Adam Raciborski, the eminent medical scientist, explained in De la puberté et de l'age critique chez la femme (1844), the increased number of women in hospitals was allowing doctors to plot accurately for the first time the menstrual cycle.[69] As noted above, the woman's cycle had traditionally been viewed as related to her fertility but the relationship had not been explained scientifically. It was acknowledged that animals were able to conceive only at certain times of the year; the question was posed whether humans were similarly restricted. In the 1840s Pouchet and Raciborski sought to provide an answer to this problem by elaborating their theory of spontaneous ovulation.[70] It had previously been believed that the sperm forced its way into the ovary, chose an egg, fertilized it, and by so doing caused it to descend. This theory had the obvious appeal that it endowed men with a freedom not enjoyed by the lower animals; the human female could be impregnated at any time. Pouchet and Raciborski argued, on the basis of their observations, however, that ovulation was spontaneous, that the egg descended independently and that fertilization, if it were to occur, could take place only at the particular time of the month when ovulation took place. Although the schedule they established was totally wrong — they stated that a woman's fertile period occurred the days just before, during, and after menstruation — the French reading public was nevertheless informed that a "natural" means of controlling conception had been discovered. Raciborski declared, "Our honorable readers will not fail to appreciate either the importance of these conclusions, or the influence that they can exercise on society from both the moral and economic point of view."[71]

The theory of spontaneous ovulation and its corollary, the rhythm method of birth control, were very quickly brought to the attention of a large reading public through the vulgarizing activities of Auguste Debay. In *Histoire des métamorphoses humaines* (1845) he announced the discovery of this new means of contraception.

> Spouses who wish to procreate must choose the four days which precede the menstrual flow or the four days which follow: spouses whose intention is not to have children will meet only after these periods. If the latter means were generally known and practiced by women, it would avoid many torments, many bitter sorrows, it would prevent many terrible consequences.[72]

The discovery of the rhythm method was a godsend, for it permitted doctors to extend legitimately their claims of expertise to include the most intimate area of human life. This is not to say that the majority of doctors now publicly defended birth control. Most did not, though what they said in the privacy of their offices is open to speculation.

What is of particular interest is the way in which those doctors who did defend birth control used this apparent advance in medical knowledge to exalt the pretensions of the profession. While extolling the rhythm method, they denigrated all other types of contraception as morally and physically dangerous. Their first argument was that it was superior to the withdrawal method because it permitted the action so necessary for the balancing of the couple's biological economy — the transmission of semen. "On the contrary [in coitus interruptus] when the function has been interrupted by a previous calculation, the erethism persists, accompanied by weakness and fatigue, and especially by a sense of sadness in which we would be tempted to see a phenomenon of the conscience similar to remorse, the first chastisement for a fault committed."[73] For an hour after such an act the result was "a collapsed state which holds the husband in a state of semi-faint." The woman was even more terribly damaged because her body had been roused to a state to expect, but then was deprived of, "la liqueur fécondante."[74] In the words of Francis Devay, "There then takes place what would happen if, showing food to a starving man, one snatched it away from his mouth, after having thus aroused his appetite." Thankfully the rhythm method permitted one to avoid such tortures: "We see . . . that science can reconcile on this point the legitimate fears of fathers of families with the laws of morality; that conjugal onanism can thus be rendered unnecessary."[75]

The second argument in favor of the rhythm method was that it was natural and so precluded both excesses and unnatural activities. Alexandre Mayer wrote, "For several years in my practice I have put to profit the knowledge of the law promulgated by M. Pouchet, with a view to turning spouses away from the vicious habits that they have adopted in their sexual activities in order not to increase their family size."[76] The rhythm method restricted sexual activity to certain periods of the month; the use of either the condom or the withdrawal method could lead to excesses at any time.

The third and most interesting argument in favor of Pouchet's method was that thanks to it, the husband could increase his control over his wife. A recurrent theme in the discussion of birth control was the fear that it would permit the woman to give free rein to her sensual desires. If the husband introduced his wife to the use of the douche, the condom, or even the withdrawal method, he was demonstrating to her how conception could be avoided. The bedroom became in the words of J.P. Dartigues an "école de démoralization," in which the shortsighted husband taught his wife how she could commit adultery without fear of detection. Such husbands "commit the stupid blunder of teaching them, on the spot, the shameful refinements of lubricity . . . [they] naturally end up by putting into practice, in their turn, with other men, the lessons that they have received from their husbands."[77] The husband who had revealed such secrets to his wife could no longer trust her. "The woman will remember, if ever her virtue is about to succumb, the lessons that she received in order to fool nature and assure her impunity, while odiously violating conjugal faith, this guardian of society."[78]

All forms of birth control would presumably provide the woman with some dangerous insights into the workings of her own body. The argument in favor of the rhythm method was based on the rather shaky premise that it maintained much of the mystery of the sexual act. Indeed, the suggestion seemed to be made that the cunning husband could keep his wife in complete ignorance of the fact that they were practicing family planning. Both procreation and contraception would continue to be the sole responsibilities of the man; the woman would remain a naive accomplice.[79]

We have seen how in the first half of the nineteenth century the French medical profession elaborated a complex argument to win the respect and confidence of bourgeois society. The doctor, in seeking to establish the status of his calling on a level equivalent to that of the church and the bar, found himself, consciously or unconsciously, assuming the role of counselor and confessor. He advanced a morality of moderation based on utility that challenged religious precepts. He promised to preserve the order and tranquility of the bourgeois household better than the priest had ever done. He assured the husband that the physician's access to the female, far from upsetting traditional mores, would increase the prerogatives of the male. He purported birth control to be the logical and final expression of medical science's ability to control the forces of both life and death. The advocacy of contraception, even by a small number of doctors, had great symbolic value. At this early date, medical science posed the most radical challenge to the moral teachings of the Catholic church.[80]

The assumption of the role of sexual censor was, of course, only one example of the general effort of the doctor to establish himself as an equal to the priest. Nevertheless, it provides the clearest example of the medical profession's claiming expertise in a field that was only peripheral to its main responsibilities and for which its specific skills and training were scarcely more sophisticated than the layman's. One of the consequences of the rise of "moral medicine" was the indefinite postponement of an objective analysis of many female complaints. Old sexual myths, now declared to be scientific truths, were given new life.[81] Women, like workers, continued to be treated as members of the congenitally unhealthy classes whose ills could only be considered worthy of attention when they threatened the smooth functioning of society. It should be stressed, however, that despite doctors' best intentions, paternal authority was inevitably undermined by medical meddling. Though physicians reiterated their desire to keep much medical knowledge secret from women, the discussion of hygiene, childbearing, and female physiology led to increased feminine conscious-ness of their bodies. The medical profession's curiously idealized and conflicting pictures of wifehood and motherhood could only contribute to such curiosity. It is striking to note, for example, that French doctors, unlike their Anglo-Saxon counterparts, rarely described women as nurturers. The state of motherhood was scarcely praised; rather it was perceived as something to be inculcated in a young woman as a moral, social, and civic duty. Discussions of the affective, spiritual benefits of motherhood were infrequent. By such omissions doctors were tacitly admitting that repeated childbearing was an excessive burden.

In later chapters we will return to the question of doctors' attitudes toward abortion and contraception at the end of the nineteenth century. When their positions were more secure, they could tackle such problems with greater confidence. But up until the 1860s they were, as we have seen, so preoccupied with the task of establishing their professional credibility that they carefully avoided public utterances that could be used to associate them with any form of contraception save that of the purported rhythm method. Their condemnations of conjugal onanism were, if anything, more terrifying than those of the priests; only the secular moralists — the subject of the following chapter — could rival physicians in the expression of populationist sentiments.

CHAPTER FOUR

Secular Moralists and Sexual Issues

Both priests and doctors had what might be called "professional interests" that led them to oppose family limitation. Equally opposed were the liberal intellectuals who in the late eighteenth and early nineteenth centuries assumed the role of secular moralists and asserted that reason, rather than religion, dictated that the questions of family, fertility, public morality, economic growth, and social reform could not be separated. The public pronouncements of philosophes, moralists, and economists on the issues of sex and population reveal the persistence, even in the writings of progressives, of traditional attitudes toward various forms of sexual behavior.

The enormous stress that the eighteenth-century philosophes placed on reason, on the necessity of man controlling his own destiny, undoubtedly played a role in justifying for some the attempt to limit family size. But many of the same writers balanced their defense of the pursuit of individual happiness with attacks on antisocial behavior. For such commentators, who in the main accepted a populationist point of view, birth control would be construed as just the kind of antisocial act that resulted from an unnatural pursuit of luxury. In 1755 Grimm asserted:

> The number of inhabitants diminishes in direct proportion to the growth of luxury; because luxury makes children burdensome to their fathers, and maintains in celibacy an infinite number of men who prefer to live comfortably and alone, than with a family which would reduce them to basic necessities. Without counting the fact that a man only thinks of marriage when he is sure of procuring and leaving to his children the same affluence which he enjoys, luxury even obliges fathers of families to take precautions against the excessive growth of their families.[1]

In *Les Intérêts de la France mal entendus* published in 1756 Ange Goudar went so far as to assert that "a certain embarrassment goes with the state of being a Husband, which is taken to the extent of making a man blush upon being united with a Spouse. . . . The women of a certain status in France find that it costs them too much to bear children; and because of this most remain spinsters, even after marriage."[2] S.N.H. Linguet rhetorically asked in a work published in 1767:

How many criminal precautions in order to prevent fecundity, without denying the pleasures which should be its reward! How many expedients in order to elude the goal of marriage, without renouncing its functions![3]

Comte L.G. Dubuat-Nançay concluded that such strategems were the first proofs that the pursuit of a life of ease and luxury was perverting sociability.

Marriage will become a fraudulent business; and if nature, always powerful, frustrates such schemes, you will hear fathers and mothers congratulate each other at the death of their children; and one will bless Heaven for this scourge, which, to be sure, will be far more common.[4]

Messance concurred in a study published just before the outbreak of the Revolution. In *Nouvelles recherches sur la population de la France* (1788) he stated what most observers of French upper-class family life had discovered: "Calculation leads a man to wish only one or two children."[5]

The physician's argument against birth control was that contraception, by freeing one from the fear of numerous offspring, encouraged sexual excesses that resulted in individual debilitation and possibly death. The secular moralist's argument was that unnatural sexual activities not only harmed the individual but undermined the relationship of the sexes, perverted the institution of the family, and threatened the very foundation of civil society.

The philosophes of the late eighteenth century and the anticlerical republicans of the nineteenth did not seek to overturn existing standards of public morality. They inveighed against sexual license with as much vehemence as did the clergy, whom they sought to rival in their pretensions to an ascetic moral code. One goal of the philosophes was to simply substitute materialism for spiritualism as the basis for ethics.[6] They advocated that the nation's institutions be judged by natural laws, and assuming that the existing patterns of bourgeois marriage and morality were natural, they set them up as a model for the rest of society. Most important, they shared the traditional fear that France faced depopulation. Indeed, the philosophes used this common concern as a stick with which to beat the privileged orders; any supposed decline in the population was attributed by them to aristocratic profligacy, fiscal injustice, or clerical celibacy. It followed that such secular moralists, anxious to prove that they were better qualified than the clergy to act as the conscience of the nation, and more concerned with the population growth of the state, would carefully avoid making any public pronouncements that might suggest their support of birth control. The question posed was not whether the individual had a right to contraception but whether or not his lack of self-discipline and social responsibility might harm the general community. The most important study of moral training to emerge in the eighteenth century was undoubtedly Rousseau's *Emile*. Rousseau expressed much the same message as Tissot. Youth was warned against the incalculable harms of solitary pleasures; the tutor was told he could never be too zealous in protecting his charge from the contamination of others and, if need be, from the child's own penchants.

> It would be very dangerous if it [instinct] taught your pupil to betray his senses and to supplement the occasions of satisfying them; once he knows this dangerous supplement he is lost. From that moment he will be forever exhausted, he will carry to the tomb itself the sad effects of this habit, the most fatal to which a young man can be subjected.[7]

As for contraception, Rousseau described it as a crime worse than the murder committed by the religious fanatic; "If irreligion does not kill men, it prevents them from being born."[8]

Tissot was one of the readers most charmed by *Emile*.[9] The two authors began to correspond in 1762. Rousseau declared that he found *L'Onanisme* a marvelous book and only regretted not having read it earlier so as to have used it as a source in his own treatment of the subject. He greeted Tissot as a comrade-in-arms in the battle for a purified morality.

> You tell me that this work [*L'Onanisme*] has been banned in Paris; this consoles me for the fact that mine [*Emile*] was burnt there; stupidity and hypocrisy, in justifying what they [the books] reprove, will reveal the shame of our species.[10]

The vogue enjoyed by works such as Tissot's was due in part to the fact that the condemnation of sexual excesses on medical grounds complemented the philosophes' attempts to use the concept of utility to justify old doctrines of moderation and continence.

> Immoderate pleasure is followed by regret, surfeit, and disgust; a passing happiness becomes a lasting misfortune. It is obvious, according to this principle, that man, who necessarily seeks happiness every moment of his life, must, when he is reasonable, keep his pleasures within bounds, refuse all those that might change into pain, and attempt to procure the most lasting happiness possible.[11]

This was the old doctrine of moderation in all things rephrased so that reason replaced obedience to God as the indicator of proper behavior.[12] Such an ideology was used to attack the "irrational" aspects of the old regime. Voltaire, for example, employed Tissot's argument against total sexual abstinence in his assault on the institution of clerical celibacy.

> In order to console this species, M. Tissot relates as many examples of illness due to retention as illnesses due to emission; and he finds these examples among women as well as among men. There is no stronger argument against the bold vows of chastity. What do you expect to become of a precious liquor, formed by nature for the propagation of the human species? If one indiscreetly wastes it, it can kill you; if one retains it, it can still kill you. It has been observed that nocturnal pollutions are often experienced by people of the two sexes who are not married, but much more often by young priests than by nuns, because the temperament of men is more dominant. One concludes from this that it is a great folly to condemn oneself to these shameful actions, and that it is a type of sacrilege by holy men to thus prostitute the gift of the Creator and to renounce marriage, expressly commanded by God himself.[13]

The philosophes sought to associate sexual abstinence with the clergy and sexual excesses with the aristocracy. The latter theme was not a new one. Even a writer such as Jean-Philippe Dutoit-Mambrini, mystic and defender of quietism, attacked contraception as but another aspect of upper-class degeneracy.[14] He published *L'Onanisme ou discours philsophiques et moral sur la luxure artificielle et sur tous les crimes relatifs* in 1760, declaring that such a book was necessary in an "impious century" that had turned its back on God. Fornication was a terrible sin, but paled to insignificance compared to the increasing practice of the *énormité secrète*. Those who wasted their seed violated both God's plan and the balance of the "animal economy." They were guilty, not only of the murder of the children they should have had, but of their children's children and so on down through the ages.[15]

> But will you avoid it [the judgment of God] and will you not also have your word in passing, new Onans, no doubt even guiltier than he. You, who without desiring to lose pleasure . . . [Dutoit-Mambrini's ellipsis] turn from its destination . . . [Dutoit-Mambrini's ellipsis] Men whose body is no less animalistic and heart no less unruly, in that the tendency is systematic; men carnally prudent, whose intentions are *that their houses shall continue forever*, as the Prophet says, *and their dwelling places to all generations* and who love to call their lands after their own names; who play with the life and existence of the children who were naturally destined to them, in limiting their number out of a concern for cupidity, prosperity, fortune, and only wish what is precisely necessary for an unmeasured and homicidal ambition.[16]

The abstinence of the poor parents of an already large household was the only form of family planning that Dutoit-Mambrini could reluctantly sanction.

> That a father and mother, poor and burdened with children, whose
> support their labor and industry can hardly provide, henceforth deprive
> themselves of one another, not out of lack of faith in the resources of
> Providence, but in order not to be inevitably a burden on society and
> charity, is perhaps not a violation of the law. [Dutoit-Mambrini adds in a
> footnote: "And yet I say this only with great suspicion of my own
> thoughts."] And it seems to me, that defensive measures taken for such
> principles are much better than continuing by a pure animality to
> produce individuals, for whom life will be onerous and hardly a benefit
> to themselves or to others.[17]

Such tolerance was not extended to the rich.

> But that opulent, rich, or well-to-do persons, without any intention of
> subduing the flesh, wish . . . without wanting to . . . [Dutoit-Mambrini's
> ellipsis] This is a crime for which our terms are reserved. Pride,
> hedonism, infamy, animality, murder, ambition, luxury, worldliness,
> distrust of Providence . . . [Dutoit-Mambrini's ellipsis] O how such
> calculators merit God to come and strike this only child, that they wish to
> raise to such a prodigious fortune, and extinguish arrangements so
> criminal.[18]

That such miscreants were not struck dead was cheerfully explained by the
author as God's way of allowing the sinful to warrant ever more frightful
punishments at the Last Judgment.

Dutoit-Mambrini claimed that his book was the first in French to
broach the subject of sexual excesses. That he presented in the vernacular
an analysis of sexual morality which had heretofore been dealt with
primarily by priests in Latin texts prepared for confessors was a sign of a
growing secular interest in such questions. His originality should not be
exaggerated, however; his condemnation of onanism, like the Catholic
clergy's, was based on the traditional premise that such an act was a
violation of God's commandment.

In the 1760s philosophes such as Diderot advanced the concept of
public utility to replace the question of morality or immorality in the
discussion of reproduction.[19] Such secular concerns were voiced as early
as 1755 by Tissot in his *Avis au peuple sur la santé*. This work was
criticized by some doctors but hailed by the philosophes as a humanitarian
undertaking destined to improve the health of the masses.[20] In the first
pages Tissot broached the population question. It was clear to him that the
countryside was being depopulated as a result of "luxe et debauche."

> Luxury obliges the rich man who wishes to cut a figure, and the man of
> middling income but the former's equal at least in every other regard,
> and who wishes to imitate him, to fear a too numerous family, whose

education will consume revenues consecrated to the expenses of appearance; and besides, if it is necessary to share his wealth among several children, they will each have very little and will be unable to maintain the standards of the father. When merit is judged by necessary expenses, one must necessarily attempt to attain and leave to one's children a situation capable of sustaining such expenses. Hence, few marriages when one is not rich; few children when one is married.[21]

It was, declared Tissot, the pursuit of the life of luxury that was causing the aristocracy to withdraw to the cities, to become idle, to indulge in debauchery, to decline in health. If and when such men did marry, they would attempt to have few children and even they would be weak and sickly.[22] Such activities were worse than sinful; they were antisocial. This new message that one was responsible to the nation even in the most intimate of activities was echoed by Moheau:

Besides, how many people are there in France today of whom the population can expect but feeble aid? How many men enervated by debauchery are decrepit in their youth; their body without vigor, their soul without desire, at the moment when this elementary fire of generation should for the first time make itself felt.[23]

The Revolution provided the *patriotes* with the opportunity to institute the regeneration of public morality sketched out by the philosophes. In C.F. Volney's *Catéchisme du citoyen,* for example, we find the same belief that the sexual activities of the individual have social ramifications.

Question: Does natural law consider as a virtue this absolute chastity so recommended in the monastic institutions?

Answer: No; because this chastity is useful neither to the society in which it takes place nor to the individual who practices it; it is even harmful to the one and the other. First, it is harmful to the society in that it deprives it of population which is one of its principal means of wealth and power and, moreover, in that bachelors, restricting their regards and affections to their life, have in general an egoism little favorable to the general interests of society. Second, it harms the individuals who practice it in that it strips them of a multitude of affections and relations which are the source of most of the domestic and social virtues; and moreover, it often happens that due to circumstances of age, diet, and temperament, absolute continence is harmful to the health and causes grave illnesses, because it violates the physical laws on which nature has founded the system of the reproduction of beings: and those who vaunt so highly their chastity, even supposing that they are acting in good faith, are contradicting their own doctrine, which consecrates that law of nature by the well-known commandment "Increase and multiply."[24]

It is not difficult to discern the impact of antionanist doctrines in such a work. Indeed, a lack of familiarity with the belief in the danger of sexual excesses would make the following passage well-nigh incomprehensible.

> Question: Does the natural law concern even the innermost desires and thoughts?

> Answer: Yes, because in the physical laws of the human body the thoughts and desires ignite the senses and soon provoke actions: moreover, by another law of nature in the organization of the body, these actions become a mechanical need which is repeated within periods of days or weeks, so that at such a moment the need for such an action, such a secretion, is reborn; if this action, this secretion, is harmful to the health, its habit will become destructive of life itself. Thus the desires and the thoughts have a true natural importance.[25]

Each succeeding regime was to have its share of moralists who warned that the social stability of the nation depended on the stamping out of the various forms of onanism. J.A. Millot and A.J. Coffin-Rosny in *Le Nestor français ou guide moral et physiologique, pour conduire la jeunesse au bonheur* referred directly to the Empire's interest in establishing stable and fruitful marriages.[26] They attributed the Revolution itself to the moral laxity of previous regimes.

> The current license of our morals is the fruit of the revolution; but the origin of their decline stems from the indecency which reigned in a segment of the works of the last century.[27]

Now more than ever before, it was necessary for youth to avoid sexual excesses. Those who indulged in such vices soon lost their vigor; more important, if such individuals in declining health did partake in fruitful intercourse, they produced sickly children. This was worse than disobeying God; it was disobeying the emperor.

> Moreover, remember that if you give in to impulses of an ardent sort too frequently, you will give to the state only individuals who, after having caused you sorrow, will be at least a burden to it. You will deserve nothing from the country for having given it a citizen, if, by your doing, he is useless to the republic in war and peace, or not fit to exploit your lands.[28]

A similar appeal to the sexual patriotism of youth was contained in P. Dusolier's *Avis aux jeunes gens des deux sexes* (1810). The Revolution had severed all moral ties; the emperor was courageously struggling to return France to order. Youth could aid in this endeavor, declared

Dusolier, by maintaining its purity and protecting its precious reserves of seminal fluid.[29]

The Restoration's campaign to restore public morality was in large part a simple continuation of the program begun by the Empire. The authorities were attempting to recreate an organic society and accordingly viewed any practice that threatened the traditional family as a danger. The clergy addressed petitions to the Penitentiary in 1816, 1822, and 1823 requesting advice on how to deal with the problem of conjugal onanism. Others turned to Tissot. Ten editions of L'Onanisme appeared between 1814 and 1830.[30]

The July Monarchy saw the public's concern for sexual morality extended from domestic to foreign policy. Lallemand declared that the most important division in the world was the one that separated the West from the lands of venereal excesses.

> After having shown the influence of monogamy and ever more severe morals on the increasing of the European populations, on their quiet, adventurous courage, on their incessant activity, on their insatiable ambition and their continued need of conquests in the sciences, the arts, industry, etc., I said that the future of the world was in the hands of the Caucasian race of the Occident. The most significant facts have come, sooner than I thought, to confirm and develop this forecast; because the explosion of the Eastern Question was only one of the practical applications of the general law discovered by observation. . . . Nothing can demonstrate in a more evident manner the power of the institutions designed to prevent semen losses: because monogamy, the moral and religious ideas adopted by all the peoples of the Occident, only act in placing an obstacle in the way of venereal excesses, which have, on the contrary, only been favored by polygamy and all the moral and religious ideas followed, in all times, in all parts, of Asia.[31]

France, having gained a base on the North African coast, was provided with yet another explanation for its actions. The providential mission of the French race — the bringing of civilization to the inactive, passive, exhausted East — was assured as long as "semen losses" were avoided.[32]

A number of schemes were hatched to combat debilitating vices on the national level. The scientist-reformer F.V. Raspail evolved a plan of combating masturbation by having all school children wear camphor-impregnated drawers. The July Monarchy's lack of interest in the scheme he attributed to political prejudice.[33] Dr. J.B.D. Demeaux offered the Second Empire an equally ambitious project. He provided an account in Mémoire sur l'onanisme of his "discovery" that masturbators were excessively shy; they particularly dreaded appearing in the nude. It followed, reasoned Demeaux, that to stamp out this vice it was simply necessary to enforce nude inspections in the schools several times a year. The effect would be to dissuade the impressionable from indulging and to discover the incorrigible by the signs of their abused bodies. But why restrict such a happy scheme to the schools? Demeaux generously envisaged his inspectors, like latter-day representatives-on-mission, fanning out across the countryside to purge the morals of the smallest hamlet.

> A small number of doctors named by the government, designated with the title of health inspectors, and charged with visiting all of France, would suffice to carry out the important mission of surveillance suggested by my scheme. . . . In a work that I have the intention of soon publishing, I hope to show that inspections, made once or twice a year in the main town of each canton, of subjects from fifteen to twenty years of age, could have the most happy results.[34]

Demeaux conceded that such an undertaking might "froiser un peu nos moeurs actuelles," but he was serenely confident that the public would recognize the utility of such measures and that the Empire would support them as part of the further advance of French civilization.[35]

The threat brandished by both doctors and moralists as the ultimate punishment of the nation that did not protect the physical health and creative powers of its males was depopulation. The association of immorality and a declining population was maintained in French minds to a surprisingly late date. As mentioned earlier, the philosophes accepted the traditional idea that France was indeed menaced by a declining birth rate. François Quesnay, convinced that agriculture was the productive sector of the economy, was as opposed as Rousseau was to those nobles whose recourse to contraception depopulated the countryside and weakened the nation both morally and physically. The new taste for luxury was again singled out as the cause of such crimes.

> Does not this dominating extravagance lead citizens to spare propagation or to avoid marriage . . . does it not induce women to seek resources in profligacy; . . . does it not remove one from labor, does it not provoke dissipation, does it not corrupt morals, does it not enervate the spirit, does it not plunge one into indolence, does it not debilitate the forces of the body?[36]

No Frenchman was to produce a Malthusian population theory in the eighteenth century.

Malthus's work appeared in French editions in 1809, 1824, 1845, and 1852. His French disciples, the liberal economists J.B. Say, Charles Ganilh, Michel Chevalier, Charles Dunoyer, and Joseph Garnier slowly won France over to the idea that a low rate of population growth was not a danger but could be taken as a sign of health.[37] In 1851 the Académie française offered a prize for the best essay on the theme that a country was fortunate when "la sagesse publique et privée" united to prevent rapid population growth. It is important to note, however, that advocating slow population growth is not necessarily the same as advocating contraception. Malthus's famous plea for "moral restraint" was aimed at convincing artisans to postpone marriage as long as possible; the parson did not condone the use of contraception and was accordingly in complete opposition to the birth controllers. As economists, not physicians, the French followers of Malthus could direct their attention to the question of why population growth should be controlled and avoid the problem of how it would be. It was not until 1863 that Joseph Garnier finally attacked Tissot for hindering the acceptance of birth control by his strictures of onanism.[38]

In this rapid survey of antionanist literature, we have attempted to give some idea of the types of argument used to oppose birth control. Secular arguments were as important as those based on religious concerns. P.J.C. Debreyne's *Essai sur la théologie* could be noted, for example, because as evidenced by its scattered references to the deaths and diseases brought on by semen losses, it is clear that the clergy had accepted the medical findings of Tissot.[39] In effect the discussion of onanism had come full circle. In the eighteenth century doctors described what they regarded as the disease of onanism in such a way that it tallied with traditional religious teachings; in the nineteenth century priests relied on the support of medical reports to back up their moral injunctions.

What is the significance of the antionanist literature? It is generally assumed that the advances made in medicine and the decline of religion created an atmosphere in which contraception could be acceptable. A study of this literature helps one to remember that numerous medical men were hostile to any sort of interference with what they chose to regard as natural functions. Moreover, the antionanist writings reveal that those indifferent to revealed religion could be as opposed as its adherents were to either masturbation or contraception on the grounds that such practices violated natural laws and were detrimental to society. Apparently, the French man or woman who turned to the physician for enlightenment on these subjects was simply warned of the dire consequences of sexual excess; what constituted "excess" was never spelled out. The blatant confusions and inconsistencies of the antionanist thesis did not seem to perturb its readers, however; they were seeking, and received, justifications for their preconceived notions. Of course, there is no way of knowing if they later refrained from either masturbation or coitus interruptus. The descriptions of the baleful diseases that accompanied onanism undoubtedly would have caused the impressionable to pause, but it is likely that others would have found the literature arousing.[40]

One of the side effects of the medical profession's condemnation of onanism was the assumption by the doctor of a position in the social hierarchy next to the priest. The growing prestige of the doctor was mainly due to the growing credibility of medical science, but the eighteenth-century physician, attempting to distinguish himself from the surgeon, who was attempting to disassociate himself from the barber, was only too eager to assume the status once monopolized by the priest — defender of public morality.[41] The public morality of France was to change very little between 1760 and 1860. Physicians, philosophes and anticlericals felt compelled to prove that a morality based on natural law was as good as, if not better than, one based on revealed religion. Their resulting moral doctrine rivaled the clergy's in its insistence on the dangers of sexual excesses. The ethics of secular France were thus basically the same as those of Catholic France, the major difference being that a new group assumed the responsibility of drawing up and defending the nation's moral code.

The argument has also been made that the diffusion of contraceptive practices reflected a growing concern for sparing women needless pain and suffering.[42] The antionanist literature would lead one to almost the opposite conclusion. It reveals that there was a widely held mental association of birth control, the "sin of Onan," and sexual excess that was a danger to health, morality, and even national prestige. Many believed that it was the *man* who was most endangered by sexual excesses; that the "demanding woman" was a menace to be viewed with mistrust.

One final lesson that can be drawn from the antionanist literature is that the historian must always be aware of the gap that separates public declarations from private practices. Despite all the morally and medically based arguments brandished by moralists and doctors, growing numbers of the French were adopting family-planning techniques. The increasing vehemence with which contraception was attacked from 1760 on was a sign not of the practice's decline, but of its growth. Balzac presented his *Deux Jeunes Mariées*, seriously discussing the necessity of limiting the number of children to two.[43] A. Bazin reported in 1833, "the bourgeois Parisian has children. He has two; no more: a girl and a boy, it was what he wanted, and 'he stopped there'. It's a phrase that he often repeats, and one to which his wife has grown accustomed."[44] In Edmond About's 1858 novel *Maître Pierre* a character replies to a questioner who asks what would happen if he should have twelve children: "Never in the wise and enlightened bourgeoisie. Twelve children maître Pierre! This unrestrained multiplication of the human species only occurs in the lower classes."[45] R.

Bruckner even had the French Malthusians make an appearance in his tale entitled *Les Intimes* (1831): "M. Duchatel, the economist has proven in a wonderful book that the poor should not have children! He is right: already young rich people have found the secret of avoiding them. Quickly put this discovery into law."[46] Indeed, by the 1830s the decline in the size of the middle-class family, complemented as it was by the popularization in France of Malthusian theories, led the socially respectable to pass increasingly over the question of the harmfulness of such practices in silence. The true heirs of the populationist sentiments of the eighteenth-century philosophes were to be the nineteenth-century socialists.

CHAPTER FIVE

Sex and Socialism:
The Opposition of the French Left
to Birth Control

The moralistic attack on family planning launched in the eighteenth century by the philosophes was continued in the nineteenth century by the socialists. Obviously the employment of contraceptive measures was taking place on such a wide scale that no serious student of social change could ignore the phenomenon; yet, at the beginning of this century Georges Sorel noted that there was no problem that socialists had treated so superficially.[1] A rapid perusal of the works of the leading nineteenth-century writers of the French left provides abundant evidence that their discussion of population pressures was not only rudimentary, it was many times confused and eccentric. In this chapter the general lines of their treatment of the population question will be sketched in and some explanations offered as to why they failed to come to grips with the problem of birth control. In isolating one problem new light will be cast on several of the broader traditions of the French left: its views on women, on the family, on pleasure — especially sexual pleasure — as a measure of happiness, and on the relationship of sex to politics.

At the start it might be objected that it is unfair to drag representatives of the French left into the courtroom of the historian and interrogate them on their ineffective analysis of an issue which at least at the start of the nineteenth century only concerned the upper and middle classes. Two responses can be made to this objection. The first is that even if birth control were in fact only practiced by the upper classes, the historian has to explain why reformers who were otherwise campaigning for full social equality should seek to prevent the lower classes from aping their "betters" in this particular area. The second is that though most observers agreed that the upper classes were the first to limit the size of their families and that the practice was then taken up in the late eighteenth century by the bourgeoisie, there were in the earliest writings on the subject references to members of the lower classes following suit. In 1760 Jean-Philippe Dutoit-Mambrini declared in *L'Onanisme* that the poor were also tempted by "defensive measures."[2] Moheau warned his readers in 1778, "Already the deadly secrets unknown to every animal but man have reached the countryside: even in the villages nature is deceived."[3] In 1782 Père Féline agreed that onanism was common among both the rich and poor.[4] By the 1850s the use of coitus interruptus by artisans had, according to Dr. Mayer, "devenu à notre époque d'un usage presque général."[5] In the latter half of the century even conservative investigators were commenting sympatheti- cally on the terror experienced by those working-class women still subjected to repeated pregnancies.

> Take a worker's wife; she prefers to be beaten than to risk having another child but; as she is the weaker, she often receives at one and the same time both the beating and the child. The fear of having a child is more frequently than one supposes a cause of discord in the poor households as well as in the wealthy.[6]

By the end of the century working-class women were demanding information on contraceptive measures. One wrote to the economist Charles Gide:

> Our poor working-class mothers see with terror the ceaseless increase of the number of their children. They cannot raise them. They often lose half of them and those left are weak and sickly. They [the mothers] are physically and morally exhausted. The great majority are ignorant of the means employed, it seems, for a long time by the well-to-do classes. . . . What they unfortunately too often do is attempt to remove the beginnings of a pregnancy. They thus injure their health. . . . In order to teach these women already overburdened with children, should we not instruct ourselves *seriously* and *honestly* [sic] on preventive measures so as to tell them of them?[7]

The responses made to such pleas by the Catholic clergy and liberal economists have been touched on. The church was hostile to birth control and true to the injunction "Go forth and multiply." The extent of family planning could not, of course, be ignored; confessors were advised to assume that it was the husband's responsibility and to avoid embarrassing questions that might drive women from the church. In the eighteenth century most French political economists accepted a growing population as a sign of the nation's well-being, but in the first half of the nineteenth century Malthus's disciples won an increasing number of converts to the theory that a stable population was preferable. Such stability was to be attained by the working class prudently postponing marriage. After France's defeat at the hands of Prussia in 1871, however, fears were expressed in terms of increasing hysteria that the country's slow population growth was leading to moral and political collapse. The century ended with the clergy and many economists rallying to ward off the threat of depopulation.[8]

What was the attitude of the French left? Its most influential representatives opposed the proposition that population could and should be controlled. Their response was motivated by the following concerns, which will be examined in detail: first, that the "population question" was a false issue manufactured by reactionaries to turn attention away from the question of social reform; second, that though population could not be controlled, nature or Providence would ensure that overpopulation would not take place; third, that if birth control freed women from their natural duties, the relationship of the sexes would be changed and the family undermined; and last, that sensual pleasure, which might be increased by the practice of birth control, was not a true measure of happiness and should not be pursued.

Considering first the left's refusal to accept the proposition that there was a "population problem," one must recall that most eighteenth-century writers believed that population growth was both a cause and an effect of a nation's wealth. Rousseau was stating a commonplace when he declared:

> What is the purpose of political association? It is the preservation and prosperity of its members. And what is the surest sign of their preservation and prosperity? It is their number and population.[9]

Indeed, the old argument that the ancient world had been more populous than the modern, and that France was actually underpopulated, was still being raised at the end of the century. Poverty, declared Mably, Morelly, and Rousseau, was not caused by the natural increase of the nation's numbers but by the faults of the existing form of society. Social inequalities could be eliminated by redistributing wealth and providing for all. The *patriotes* carried on this argument into the Revolution, attributing what they took to be a declining population to fiscal injustices and ecclesiastical celibacy. François-Noël Babeuf, the heir of the Spartan egalitarianism of Rousseau and Mably, who made the first practical attempt at establishing a socialist state, set the line of the nineteenth-century socialists' discussion of population. Population pressure did not pose a problem to existing society; if it were to in the future, it still could only be considered a secondary issue.

> I believe that even in the case where it was recognized that the means of subsistence of a Nation would not be sufficient to satisfy the appetites of all its members; I believe that then the simple laws of nature command, instead of depopulation, the partial deprivation of each of its members, to satisfy equally, in the usual proportions the needs of all.[10]

Babeuf was addressing himself to a hypothetical case, but his concern reflected the spirit of the times; a year after his death in 1798 Malthus published what was to be the most famous study of the problem, *An Essay on the Principles of Population.*

Malthus was not a disinterested observer; he undertook his investigations with the purpose in mind of destroying the egalitarian theories of Godwin and Condorcet. The result of such utopian schemes, declared Malthus, would be that population would soon overshoot the food supply and be overwhelmed by vice and misery. For his contemporaries his most startling revelation, however, was not that food supplies were increasing in arithmetic progression and population in geometric progression, but that the major cause of existing poverty was the "reckless over-breeding of the poor."[11] The upper classes in both France and England, slowly having to relinquish traditional arguments for the maintenance of their privileged status, were now provided with modern, scientific justifications. Malthus had proven to their satisfaction that reform was futile.

After Malthus French liberal economists swung round to the view that an ever-increasing population was not desirable. Writers on the left who quite naturally viewed Malthus as an advocate of the propertied classes clung to the older opinion that the failure of a nation to grow had to be seen as a sign of decay; such growth could be more than made up for by the increases in productivity provided by organized labor. Henri Saint-Simon, considered a man of the left to the extent that he was opposed to individualistic capitalism, was true to the spirit of the eighteenth century in declaring population growth the best test of a country's prosperity.[12] His early associate Auguste Comte described population as the mother of social progress and decried Malthus's argument as a sophistic theory, an amalgam of "irrational exaggerations," an immoral aberration which revealed the antipathy of the wealthy for the poor.[13] Philippe-Michel Buonarroti, who popularized Babeuf's thought in the *Conspiration pour l'égalité* (1828), carried on the master's message that in the egalitarian state everything would "favor the multiplication of the species."[14] In *Voyage en Icarie* (1840) the communist Étienne Cabet claimed that in his reformed society the population would be doubled.[15] P.J. Proudhon, though critical of every other contemporary socialist, did agree that Malthus was responsible for the propagation of a doctrine that would destroy both the family and the economy.

> The family dies out and with the family property; the economic movement is left unfinished, and society returns to a state of barbarism. Malthus and the moral economists made marriage inaccessible; the physician-economists make it purposeless: both add to the lack of bread the lack of affections, provoke the disintegration of social ties.[16]

The romantic socialist Pierre Leroux was of the same opinion; the "population question" was simply another attack launched by liberals on the lower classes.

> After having preached to the poor continence, celibacy, and forbidden marriage before the age of thirty, they have invented what they call *checks* or artificial obstacles to population. . . . To teach men to satisfy their instincts without obeying the laws of nature, to violate them, was a shame reserved for the atheists that are called economists.[17]

In England, wrote Leroux, the same economists, ignorant of both the moral and economic calamities that declining population produced, were going so far as to defend infanticide.[18]

Now it is important to recall that Malthus's famous plea for "moral restraint" was aimed at convincing the poor to postpone marriage as long as possible; the parson did not condone the use of contraception after marriage and was thus in complete opposition to the birth controllers. This nuance in Malthusian thought was overlooked by many of his disciples and critics. Both sides were far more concerned with his major argument that individual self-improvement and social reform were mutually exclusive, antagonistic goals. In adopting this premise the Left had no choice but to oppose population control; to accept the social necessity of either contraception or postponed marriage would, it was felt, be tantamount to acknowledging that unemployment and poverty were natural problems to be overcome by individual self-help.

When the left suspected anyone who worried about the population problem of being an enemy of social reform, did this mean that they foresaw the population increasing interminably? Such a proposition, they recognized, was untenable. They were thus led to elaborate the second theme of their anti-Malthusian argument, that once a socialist society was created the population would be balanced by "natural means."[19] Just as a man stops growing once he reaches maturity, so too would the population cease to increase once society reached some predetermined level of development. A problem arose, however, when the various socialist theorists attempted to explain the means by which benevolent nature would prevent overpopulation from occurring.

Proudhon condemned contraception and declared that abortion, defended by someone he referred to as a certain Dr. G . . . , was equal to murder. Charles Loudon's theory that population stability could be attained by extending a mother's period of lactation, during which she was less fertile (a theory that won Leroux's interest), was also rejected by Proudhon on the grounds that it sprang from a pessimistic appraisal of man's potential.[20] Even the rhythm method, which involved no artificial checks to offend the susceptibilities of the natural law advocate, was declared to be morally unacceptable.

> With this easy means of playing without paying, and of sinning without being surprised, modesty is no longer but a stupid and troublesome prejudice, marriage a bothersome and useless convention.[21]

It was the very idea that birth control made life easier for man that most enraged Proudhon. Labor was the essential characteristic of the human being; struggle and sacrifice of pleasure produced progress. The limitation of population could thus be viewed only as a sign of moral advance if it were a consequence not of the pursuit of pleasure but of a greater devotion to labor. Proudhon claimed, as had Comte, that the great men of history had led chaste lives while the lazy and poor had been prolific. This was the real law of population.

> The industrial faculty exercises itself only at the expense of the prolific faculty. Labor is an active cause of the cooling of love: it is the most powerful of all antiaphrodisiacs, that much more powerful especially as it simultaneously affects the mind and the body.[22]

The argument of the socialist theoretician Louis Blanc was similar to Proudhon's in that it contained the idea that the cultivation of manners, the displacement of the lower appetites by the higher, would have a depressing effect on the birth rate.[23] He declared that natality was simply a reflection of the standard of living; when the latter reached a certain level, smaller families would become the norm. To support his thesis he presented data drawn from Paris which revealed that the wealthier *arrondissements* had fewer births per family than the poorer.[24] The question was to be asked, however, why England, which was more prosperous than France, continued to have a faster growing population.

The discussion of the natural leveling-off of population led even Louis-Auguste Blanqui, traditionally portrayed as the cool, calculating revolutionary, into realms of bizarre speculation. He shared Blanc's belief that as the standard of living was raised the birth rate dropped, but he interpreted this phenomenon in a most peculiar fashion. The improvements in public health that would inevitably follow the Revolution would result in a preponderance of male births. With fewer women there would be smaller population increases, although each mother would still bear a large number of children. The *faits connus* on which Blanqui based his theory were drawn from contemporary reports on Tibet.[25] Setting aside the exotic trappings of the argument, one can see that Blanqui's response to the birth control issue was essentially the same as that of most other socialists — a refusal to envisage the direct control of conception as either moral or natural and a faith in Providence eventually providing a panacea. The antithesis of the class struggle and individual self-help was reiterated. After the Revolution a real solution to the population problem would be provided not just for calculating individuals but for all.[26]

The third theme of the French left's argument against birth control was that it was immoral, inasmuch as the practice violated not divine but natural laws. By freeing women from their natural duties and responsibilities, it frustrated the purposes of the family and threatened society at large. Here again nineteenth-century social theorists were following their eighteenth-century forebears. The philosophes had sought not to tear down but to build up society on surer foundations. Though they criticized ethics based on religious values, they insisted that their natural morality would provide a guarantee of public order. The family, in the eyes of such men, was the source of all social cohesion, a natural entity that had to be buttressed, not undermined. Morelly, for example, believed that by marrying and having children a man provided evidence of his interest in the well-being of the community and therefore, in his *Code de la nature* (1755), marriage was made obligatory.[27] It was due to this concern for the family unit that the philosophes who, save for Condorcet, were otherwise little interested in women, felt forced to devote some attention to the role of wife and mother. There was always the danger, warned Rousseau, that the weaker sex, in giving in to its natural penchant for indolence and licentiousness by refraining from having children, could undermine both the family and the state.

> Since the state of motherhood is onerous, one soon finds the means of avoiding it altogether; one wishes to do a useless task [i.e., have sex but avoid conception] in order to continually redo it, and to the detriment of the species is turned the attraction given in order to multiply it.[28]

Similarly, Babeuf viewed women with their more passionate natures as a threat to the communist society he envisaged, in which happiness would be found not in sensual pleasure but in hard work.[29] Future harmony, he declared, would depend on limiting their education, maintaining their domestic subordination, and dulling their senses by manual labor. According to Buonarroti, however, women's work was not to interfere with their primary function: "The man, destined by nature to [a life of] movement and action, must feed and defend the country; the woman must give it vigorous citizens."[30] Cabet was working toward the same sort of state in which marriage and fidelity would be civic duties. Celibacy and adultery were to be crimes in Icarie; the moral control of the community would in addition preclude youth from having any "secrets." Cabet, instead of discussing birth control, presented a plan for both the doubling of the population and the breeding of a super race. Woman was not to be freed from childbearing; she was to be subjected to the dictates of a *Commission de perfectionnement.*[31]

A radical change in the appreciation of women has been credited by a number of historians to Saint-Simon and his ilk.[32] Saint-Simon himself showed little real interest in improving the status of women. His follower Barthélemy-Prosper Enfantin preached the "rehabilitation of the flesh," but it is difficult to determine what his heralded emancipation of women meant in practical terms.[33] In theory he broke down the old laws of matrimony; in practice he and his followers attempted to prove their higher morality by leading an ascetic life at Ménilmontant. Enfantin, his time taken up as it was by the more serious business of searching for the "Woman Messiah," had no time for such mundane problems as birth control and does not seem to have considered the population problem. Far from freeing woman, he envisaged subjecting both sexes to the theocratic rule of the *Mère* and *Père.*

Enfantin's religious mysticism represented one aspect of Saint-Simon's patrimony; Auguste Comte's positivism, another.[34] The church had presented woman as primarily a propagator of the species; Comte declared that her essential vocation was that of wife. This was hardly emancipation. Wife and husband were not equal; man was superior in force, woman in affection. Comte condemned the "subversive dreams" of the feminists and restricted the wife to her "august domestic vocations." Seclusion was necessary because men and women could only be friends if they were not competitors. The woman, wrote Comte, was to renounce all power and become the priestess of humanity, representing by her abnegation the subordination of politics to morality.

In Comte's writings one finds the same puritanical streak noted earlier in Babeuf and Cabet. Marriage was for Comte the basic relationship of society and, accordingly, had to be monogamous and indissoluble. The purpose of the marriage was to purge the couple's love of all base passions. Though Comte loathed Malthus, he downplayed the woman's role as childbearer. Sexual desire was, he admitted, necessary first to bring the couple together, but from that point on this instinct was to be subjected to a "constant and severe discipline" leading to "conjugal chastity."[35]

A remarkably similar aversion to sexuality is found in the works of Proudhon, who brought together all the misogynist arguments of the century. Woman, in his eyes, was inferior to man physically, intellectually, and morally, existing somewhere between him and the animal world.[36] Once her childbearing function was completed she lost even this position and became a *sorte de métis.*[37] Men and women were, he declared, two distinct species who could form no true society. The only time they came together was during sexual intercourse — an unfortunate duty required for the continuation of the species. It was during these brief encounters, however, that man ran the danger of falling completely under ths sway of woman and the sensual desires she incarnated. He was only saved from this fate by the fact that nature had condemned woman to pay a terrible physical price for her brutish lusts.

> Rousseau was mistaken, in counseling the married woman to be prudent and discreet in her relations with her husband. A woman never says: "Enough!" It is up to the man to take his own counsel and not exhaust himself. Certainly, the modest, reserved woman who refuses out of tenderness, out of foresight, out of respect for her husband and herself, this woman is a divine idea; but she is not a reality. The reality is just the opposite. It is up to the man to contain himself, and to be always grave, severe; if not, his wife, knowing his weakness, will deride him and devour him.
> Man, with his force, his will, his courage, his intelligence, daily falling into the amorous traps of the woman, would never succeed in taming her and making himself master if he were not aided by the maladies and infirmities which beat down this lioness: pregnancies, births, nursings, then all the diseases which follow and permit the man, in withdrawing from the common bed to catch his breath and become himself again, while the woman, beaten down by suffering, is constrained to bow and humble herself; there is the source of domestic peace.[38]

Michelet had also described the woman as a permanent invalid;[39] what he did not appreciate, declared Proudhon, was that only by her physical incapacitation could man be free. Her passions had to be bridled by physical suffering if the family were to play its role of providing the dignity, pious calm, and moral sentiment previously furnished by religion. Birth control, which provided the woman with a way of avoiding the consequences of concupiscence, was thus necessarily viewed by Proudhon as posing the gravest possible threat to the social order.

> Pornocracy [Proudhon's term for female emancipation] and Malthusianism must go together. They appeal to one another, they join, unite, harmonize, as cause and effect. One asks that no more children be produced and the other teaches how to have no more than: Polyandry for women. Polygamy for men. Promiscuity for all.[40]

Proudhon was the one major figure on the French left to win a reputation as an unabashed misogynist. It has been assumed by historians that aside from this renegade all nineteenth-century socialists can be classified as feminists to the extent that they envisaged a better future for women.[41] But it was this tendency of the utopian socialists to discuss the state of motherhood only as it would be after the ultimate social transformation that often blinded them to the very real problems posed by childbearing to nineteenth-century women. The chilling description of the plight of the working-class mother in *De la répartition des richesses* (1846), the work of the Fourierist François Vidal, provides a useful corrective to contemporary effusions on the joys of motherhood.

> The towers [of the foundling homes] have been closed, and the poor mother, the working-class girl, has been left no other option than abortion or infanticide. In our bleak society many mothers have cursed their fecundity, and more than one, in thinking of the future which awaits her newborn child, has broken its head against the cobbles, or strangled it with maternal hands, in order *to deliver it from life*, to spare it misery, suffering, to save it from prostitution. Happy those children of the working class who die in the cradle! Happy the sterile woman! Happy the man with no family![42]

But even Vidal, who bitterly portrayed the burden of motherhood in the somberest of tones, did not suggest that an answer was provided by birth control. He, too, believed that there was only one way to prevent the horrible act of infanticide and that was by the wholesale changing of society. His unstated assumption, shared by most other socialists, was that if society provided the necessary means of support, women could be expected to accept uncomplainingly pregnancy after pregnancy.

The fact that many writers on the left denied that the sensual pleasure of either the woman or the man could be taken as a true measure of happiness was a final reason for their rejection of birth control. At bottom these writers shared the traditional moralists' pessimistic conception of humanity. Like them they believed that social cohesion could only be attained by the individual's sacrifice of pleasure. Man had to choose either the frugality and simplicity of the ascetic or the decadence and degeneration of the sensualist.[43]

The consequences of the sexual overindulgence which contraceptive practices would permit included both physical and moral debility. As the following passage from Leroux makes clear, it was assumed that to free sexual gratification from the consequences of conception would inevitably lead to debauchery.

> Do they imagine that they can create, as they counsel, *checks* on the population, without burdening Humanity with evils of all sorts, without afflicting it with every vice, without imposing on it every type of impurity, without making human life an eternal hell![44]

These "checks" would permit promiscuous liaisons before marriage to go undetected and allow sexual excesses during marriage. The doctors P.J.B.

Buchez and U. Trélat in the midst of their participation in the Carbonari and Saint-Simonian movements warned the young man, "But if, on the contrary, he delivers himself to hasty pleasures, he will ruin his constitution, will remain sickly and weak, lose his memory, his will, and use up his life in a few moments."[45] Sexual excess within marriage was defined by the authors as anything more than intercourse twice a week. Moreover, it was the man's responsibility to protect the physical and moral health of the family; one could not expect wives to have such foresight. "Coition is infinitely less tiring for them than for the man, they can repeat it with impunity."[46] Women were more sensitive but less sensible creatures, wholly dominated by their sexual desires and therefore a real threat to their husbands' welfare.

The question of preserving one's physical health was only a secondary consideration; the moral consequences of the sensual excesses permitted by birth control were the socialists' real concern. Proudhon was sounding a familiar chord when he declared that it was by shunning pleasure and devoting himself to work that man demonstrated his humanity.

> This antagonism of the physical and moral in man, in the exercise of his industrial and prolific faculties, is the balance wheel of the social machine. Man, in his development, moves ceaselessly from fatality to liberty, from instinct to reason, from matter to spirit. It is by virtue of this progress that he frees himself little by little from the slavery of the senses, as from the oppression of painful and repulsive labors.[47]

Man had to flee "the tyranny of the organs" and seek in marriage a chaste love that would vanquish the passions. Proudhon was in effect saying that the coming of a reformed society would entail as much a moral as an economic and political revolution. "Either humanity must become by labor a society of saints, or by monopoly and misery civilization is only a vast orgy."[48]

Half a century later Georges Sorel was voicing the same sentiments. He hailed Proudhon as the defender of morality based on family and sexual relations; he ridiculed the feminist programs of Fourier and Bebel. Yet Sorel recognized that women were not happy with their lot.

> But it is necessary never to forget that the woman is the great regulator of birth and that everywhere, as soon as she is no longer raised in the superstitious respect of the force of the male, she demands the right of not being transformed into a reproductive animal.[49]

The problem, as Sorel saw it, was how to relieve women of this burden without releasing the destructive forces of sexuality. Like Comte he insisted that the woman not be dragged down to the man's level by giving her rights to "caprices amoureux." Like Proudhon he insisted that the answer was to be found in greater chastity for all: "We can affirm that *the world will become more just only to the extent that it becomes more chaste*; I do not believe that there is a more certain truth."[50]

Why did the major writers on the left attack the idea of birth control as unnatural, immoral, and impolitic? The first point to be made is that they were not alone in inadequately dealing with the question of contraception. Alfred Naquet, the "father of divorce," was referring to every political following when he asked in 1901, why, despite the fact that birth control was practiced on such a wide scale, no one dared to defend it.[51] The socialists' writings on the subject were, of course, prescriptive, not descriptive. It is difficult to determine when authors were seriously condemning specific practices and when they were striking moralistic poses. Even Paris doctors, whose families in the 1890s averaged, one authority informs us, 1.5 children, were extremely circumspect when it came to discussing birth control in public. Their references to the practice were more often designed to alarm than to enlighten. "L'onanisme conjugal, fléau plus cruel, plus meutrier, plus épouvantable que le typhus, la peste et le choléra réunis."[52]

Though the decline of the birth rate was noted with anxiety from the 1850s on by a host of social observers, there were few who chose to regard it as a consequence of simple family planning. Most attributed the decline to whatever aspect of contemporary society they considered most noxious and therefore most likely to result in sterility. The list included conscription, capitalism, clerical celibacy, urbanization, secularization, taxation, equal inheritance, freemasonry, overeating, bicycling, alcoholism, absinthe, tobacco, and both the emancipation and subjugation of women.

But, in explaining the response of the left to the challenge of birth control, it is not sufficient to state simply that they shared the prudishness of their contemporaries. Equally important was their sensitivity to the conservatives' charge that they were propagating immoral doctrines. The vociferousness with which socialists insisted on their moral superiority suggests that many felt constrained to buttress moral norms in order to compensate for their social critiques. They were so concerned to prove that their economic reforms would not lead, as their opponents claimed, to social disintegration that they defended the patriarchal family, advocated the subordination of women, and condemned any change in the relationship of the sexes as unnatural. Proclaiming, as had traditional moralists, that social cohesion was achieved by the individual's sacrifice of pleasure, they could then view birth control as a highly individualistic act prompted by self-interest and contempt for the community.

An analysis of the fertility debate, as the last four chapters has established, provides a way of setting aside the time-honored but superficial political antagonisms of the nineteenth-century French moralists and of isolating their more basic but less frequently acknowledged common concerns. The left did not break with traditional Judeo-Christian morality. Only a few writers were to declare that sexual and political repression were related; and an even smaller number accepted the notion that the freedom of women to control their own bodies was an essential liberty. By 1860 the subject of "sexual politics" had only been broached; the full debate had to await the appearance of Paul Robin.

PART THREE

The Critics

CHAPTER SIX

Paul Robin

By the latter decades of the eighteenth century the restriction of family size was a well-established custom among the nobility, and by the first decades of the nineteenth century the bourgeoisie and peasantry were following suit. The general acceptance of such practices by the propertied to protect their patrimony did not lead, however, to any public defense of the individual's right to contraception. On the contrary, as shown in the previous section, the view prevailed that both women and urban workers risked being debauched if they had easy access to such information. As a consequence the curious situation arose that it required the active engagement of a revolutionary, imbued with socialist and feminist sympathies with the belief that women and workers could not be left in ignorance of their rights to control fertility, to launch the birth control campaign in France. This man was Paul Robin. In 1878 Robin produced the first French work devoted to the defense of fertility control. But it was more than this; it was also an attempt to place the limitation of the size of the working-class family into a political context. The work thus shocked Malthusian economists because of its radicalism while it offended socialists because it linked sex and politics. *La Question sexuelle* began with the ringing appeal:

> Oh, you who are called proletarians (that is to say, *makers of children*), you who are crushed by an excess of labor, you who are poorly housed, badly dressed, poorly fed, if you sense your pains, if you aspire to things the possession of which would permit you to struggle against the tyranny so well organized by your oppressors, do not burden yourself with a *great number* of beings more feeble, more powerless than you! Do not encumber yourself with children! . . . Such prudence is as desirable in the daily industrial battle as it is in the violent struggle of the day, very close at hand I hope, of the social revolution.[1]

Paul Robin, born in 1837 in Toulon, began his public life as a teacher in provincial *lycées* but moved quickly, inspired by positivist and socialist leanings into revolutionary politics during the Second Empire.[2] Forced to abandon both France and his profession, he founded in Brussels with Cesar de Paepe and Eugène Hins the *Association positiviste*. At the same time he entered the International Working Men's Association. It was because of his involvement with the I.W.M.A. that upon his return to France in 1870 he was arrested and again exiled, this time to England. All his life Robin was to prove to be an irritable, difficult man to work with, partly because of the originality of his ideas. After having quarreled with Bakunin and his followers on the continent, Robin later found himself equally at odds with Marx and his adherents in London. Marx expelled Robin from the executive of the International in 1871, and he thus found himself effectively cut off from any future political activity. It was in this frame of mind that he turned to the study of Malthusian economics. In London a Malthusian League was in the process of being set up by the Drysdale family.[3] Malthus had warned of the dangers of overpopulation but opposed birth control. The members of the League, espousing what would be known as neo-Malthusianism, revised the master's message; according to them, it was futile to expect wide-scale abstinence, and therefore only by an artificial restriction of family size could the working class hope to assure its prosperity. The League thus sought to fuse its socially conservative economic views with a popular appeal for fertility control. Although the League (thanks to the patronage of the Drysdales), was to be kept in existence for over fifty years, it was doomed to failure. The English working classes, at whom its veiled appeals for fertility control were aimed, could not help but be alienated by a doctrine asserting that the poverty they endured was due not to the failings of the social system but to their own fecklessness.

The Malthusian League was singularly unsuccessful at home, but it did prove capable of interesting foreign observers in the population question. This was no doubt due in part to the fact that it was tolerant of continental socialists because their theorizing posed no direct challenge to English society. The Drysdales' most important convert, a disciple who was to turn the neo-Malthusian message to his own purposes, was Paul Robin. Convinced that birth control complemented the revolutionary struggle, in 1877 he tried to win the support of the anarchist congress at Saint-Imier to his new belief; he was rebuffed.[4] He then produced an appeal intended for the 1879 congress of socialists at Marseilles. It was in this way that *La Question sexuelle* was produced, which after revisions appeared as a brochure entitled *Le Secret de bonheur*. But in the 1880s Robin had to rein in his enthusiasm for birth control propaganda. Permitted to return to France by the republican government, he was entrusted by the Ministry of Education, now dominated by anticlericals, with the supervision of an orphanage at Cempuis. Clearly, it would have been imprudent for the director of such an establishment to be known to the public as a sex radical. In any event Robin's nomination to the post was a provocative move in itself. During his years in the International Working Men's Association he had defended the principles of coeducation, the mix of theoretical and practical training known as "integral education," and positivist morality; at Cempuis he attempted to put this mélange of ideas into practice. Robin was in later years to be hailed as one of the most important socialist theoreticians of education. In this study it is only possible to note that his pedagogical views harmonized with his ideas on population inasmuch as both were founded on the central belief in the rights of the individual to self-control.[5]

In the 1880s Robin surreptitiously kept up his birth control activities. He visited London for the Malthusian League Conference in 1884 and had Charles Drysdale visit his orphanage in the same year; he used the Cempuis presses to run off copies of *Le Secret de bonheur* and in 1889 opened a Paris dispensary to provide women with contraceptives.[6] There was some talk of these ventures in the press, but it was primarily due to his anticlericalism and defense of coeducation that conservatives succeeded in 1894, during the wave of repression against the anarchist outrages, in driving him from his post.[7] Robin later claimed to have been relieved that his newfound freedom permitted him to plunge fully into the fertility debate. He assumed that the time was now ripe for a French version of the Malthusian League; a Dutch neo-Malthusian League had been established in 1885 and a German movement in 1889. Robin himself avoided direct references to Malthus when he christened his own 1896 organization the Ligue de la régénération humaine. It had only a small handful of adherents and those it drew mainly from the ranks of the syndicalist and libertarian left.[8]

The Ligue's first actions were to distribute a birth control tract translated from the Dutch, *Moyens d'éviter les grandes familles*, and to set up a journal entitled *Régénération*. Robin himself made direct appeals to doctors, scientists, and politicians for support. Little was forthcomng. Instead, questions were asked in the Assembly about the possible criminality of the Ligue's actions. The popular press expressed its outrage. *Le Figaro* noted that the cartoonist Willette had been prosecuted for a mere caricature and asked why Robin was not then tried for his "criminal and immoral propaganda." *Le Temps* accused him of masquerading as a respectable social observer while undermining the nation, and *La République française* attacked the "homme de Cempuis" for indulging in bizarre and extravagant theorizing that could only weaken the social fabric.[9] Clearly surprised by the violence of the attack, Robin foolishly responded by referring to the government as being made up of killers and impostors. Threatened with a jail term for his outburst, he fled to London, from which he launched a counterblast, "Aux richards et aux hommes de lettres."[10] In the tract he attributed his persecution to the populators and their "stupid fear of a foreign invasion, and especially, though they do not say it, their terror of the demands of exploited workers."[11] In failing health Robin decided to remove himself even further from the area of conflict, and in August of 1898 he set sail for New Zealand. For ten months he was befriended by A.W. Bickerton, professor of chemistry and physics at Canterbury College, who at Wainomi had established a commune of sorts called the "Federated Home." Bickerton was a feminist interested in questions of fertility control and appears to have provided Robin with additional information on contraception.[12]

Back in France the journal *Régénération* disappeared, but the Ligue did gain the support of one or two radical publications such as *La Fronde* and *Les Droits de l'homme* as well as the adhesion of personalities such as Dr. Adrien Meslier, Mason, socialist and future deputy for Paris (1902–1914), J.B. Clément, anarchist poet and editor of the *Petit République*, and Eugène Fourniére, socialist deputy for the Aisne (1898–1902). Assured that he would not be prosecuted, Robin returned to Paris in July of 1899, reestablished the Ligue and began again in April of 1900 the publication of *Régénération*. Slowly but surely the organization built up its support during the next eight years.[13] In fact the Ligue prospered due to its sale of contraceptives and sex manuals. As a result, when a falling-out occurred among the leadership in 1908, with Robin being opposed for his dogmatism by Albert Gros and Eugène Humbert, the movement was not weakened but went on from strength to strength. Gros founded *Le Malthusien* and Humbert *Génération consciente*. Robin, now in his seventies, withdrew from active work, cantankerous as ever, but at least content in the knowledge that he had firmly established a place for the topic of birth control in the population debate.

Why did the defense of birth control in France become the monopoly of left-wing libertarians such as Paul Robin? To understand how Robin concocted his particular defense of fertility control, it is necessary to disentangle the strands of thought from which it was woven — Malthusian population concerns, eugenic fears, feminist sympathies, and socialist interests. First, it must be noted that given the pronatalist disposition of economists both on the left and right, Malthus's population doctrines were never to win great support in France.[14] In the first half of the nineteenth century J.B. Say, Joseph Garnier, and Charles Dunoyer did what they could to make the Englishman's doctrine of the need to limit population growth acceptable to French audiences.[15] They did not, however, compromise their respectability by defending the artificial restriction of family size. Given the low rate of population growth already evident in France by mid-century, it could have been concluded that explicit directions were not needed. Indeed, some congratulated themselves on the fact that France was proving the hypotheses of Herbert Spencer and Auguste Comte that a decline in fertility was a natural concomitant of a growth in civilization; as nervous energy was switched from reproductive to cultural purposes family size would naturally shrink.[16] The working classes, being less "civilized," however, did need to have drawn to their attention the dangers of indulging unthinkingly in pursuit of pleasure. Such, for example, was the burden of a Malthusian work entitled *Manuel de morale et d'économie politique à l'usage des classes ouvrières* written in 1853 by J.J. Rapet. In this novelistic treatment of social and economic problems, Rapet, following Harriet Martineau, presented a picture of workers being enlightened to the wonders of political economy. The hero of the tale, a doctor Dupré, overcomes the ignorance and suspicion of villagers by helping them establish schools, build roads, and recognize the artificiality of class conflict. Poverty is presented as a personal problem to be overcome by the worker avoiding the café, saving at the *caisse d'épargne*, and following the "prudence" of the upper classes in marrying late in life.

> Now, [asks Dupré] whose responsibility is it if there are few or many factory hands? It is not the masters' but really the workers'. Let the workers marry prudently and they will not end up with a horde of children whom they cannot raise or only raise for their own misfortune; and in waiting, live chaste, sober, active, and thrifty lives. Let them prepare themselves to one day taste the joys of fatherhood without having to fear the cruelest torment, that of not being able to feed their children
>
> — Thank you, Monsieur Dupré, said many workers, we will follow your advice.[17]

That such a hackneyed account of laissez-faire economics would have won the attention of many workers seems most unlikely, but it was a sign of the times that the book was a prize winner of the Académie des sciences morales et politiques. It was just this sort of moral tale that continued to be employed by the Malthusian League in England well into the twentieth century. In France, however, fears of depopulation compounded by the growth of a powerful Germany after 1870 led to Malthusian doctrines being attacked from all sides. Frédéric Bastiat, Paul Leroy-Beaulieu, Daniel Villey, Charles Gide, and others took up the cry that falling fertility was not some innocent side effect of a growth of civilization but a symptom of social malaise.

It is noteworthy that Paul Robin was educating himself in Malthusian doctrines while in exile in London, in the very decade in which the depopulationist fears were given full vent in France. As a result, when he returned to Paris in the 1880s, he brought with him doctrines that, though they might have appeared shocking in the 1860s, now appeared positively traitorous. Anglo-Saxon influence was to be important in much of the early French birth control literature. But the earliest birth control propagandists asserted that their ideas were based on French practices. Francis Place claimed in 1823 that Robert Owen visited France for the purpose of informing himself on means of contraception.[18] Robert Dale Owen asserted in *Moral Physiology* (1830) that the French had proved the harmlessness of contraception:

> What the experience of the French nation positively proves, [is] that man may have a perfect control over this instinct; and that men and women may, without any injury to health, or the slightest violence done to the moral feelings, and with but small diminution of the pleasure which accompanies the gratification of the instinct, refrain at will from becoming parents.[19]

And having drawn their lessons from France the Anglo-Saxon writers in a sense returned the favor by providing the French with texts on contraception. George Drysdale's *Physical, Sexual and Natural Religion* (1855) appeared in French as *Les éléments de science sociale* (1869), Henry Allbutt's *The Wife's Handbook* (1885) as *Le livre de l'épouse* (1898) with an introduction by Dr. Lutaud, and Charles Knowlton's *Fruits of Philosophy* (1832) as *Plus d'avortements!* (1899). The leader of the English Malthusian League, Charles Drysdale, directed much of the neo-Malthusian proselytizing in France. When the *Gazette médical de Paris* was stimulated by the appearance in 1878 of the Malthusian League to comment that the movement's task was hopeless because it was impossible to prevent people from having children, Drysdale promptly replied that a glance at the size of middle-class families — especially those of doctors — proved that this was not the case. They clearly practiced onanism, which the Bible might castigate, but which the scientific had to applaud.[20]

It was Drysdale's intention to recruit as much medical support as possible, and he accordingly attended the 1879 Medical Congress in Amsterdam, from which he reported that Dr. Leblond of Paris stated that conjugal prudence was not harmful and Dr. Lutaud confirmed his suspicions that most French physicians practiced coitus interruptus. Drysdale prevailed upon both to join the Malthusian League's Medical Branch and was also successful in having the economist Yves Guyot and the deputy M. Talandier accept posts as vice-presidents of the organization.[21] What Drysdale could not obtain was the *active* support of these men for birth control propaganda *within* France. Having one's name

listed as a corresponding member of a foreign organization dedicated to
the discussion of population problems was one thing; publicly declaring
oneself an adherent of unpopular views at home was another.[22] Drysdale
thus found the neo-Malthusian message propounded in France, not by
respectable physicians or social scientists, but by the well-known
subversive Paul Robin.

Robin clearly stated in tracts such as *Malthus et les néo-Malthusiens*
(1905) that while he accepted Malthus's contention that pressure of
population could contribute to the cause of poverty, it was the social
system itself which had to be changed. Whereas the English
neo-Malthusians presented birth control as a means by which the poor
could adjust to the demands of the capitalist economy, Robin presented it
as a measure by which they could prepare themselves for its overthrow.
He recognized that Malthus had not undertaken his investigations as a
disinterested observer but as one determined to destroy the utopian
schemes of Godwin and Condorcet. Working-class suspicions of
population discussions were therefore warranted. Robin cited as an
example the popular poem of Pierre Dupont which included the lines:

> Suivons le peuple et sa science
> Sifflons Malthus et ses arrêts![23]

What the working class had to be told was that birth control, though not a
panacea, was a tactic that could be turned to their own purposes. Priests,
economists, and even doctors attempted to keep the working class
ignorant of their own physiology; some socialists refused to acknowledge
the short-term benefits of small families. The real friends of labor would
help in the diffusion of contraceptive information so needed by
working-class women. Robin was clearly a Malthusian of sorts, but his
interests were obviously far removed from the conservatism of both the
orthodox Malthusians in France or the neo-Malthusians in England.

A second element clearly discernible in Robin's defense of birth
control were his vague eugenic concerns. The hope that the rational
control of fertility could aid in the improvement of the race was implied in
the title Robin gave his organization — Ligue de la régénération humaine.
Even his earlier educational activities revealed how much he had been
marked by his scientific interest in Darwin and Comte. At Cempuis
he kept careful anthropometric records on his charges, at the same time
allowing them every freedom. In a curious way he thus manifested a
hankering after positivistic certainties combined with a love for Fourierist
spontaneity.[24] This same tension could be found in his defense of birth
control. On the one hand he defended contraception on libertarian

grounds, but on the other he spoke of the *duty* of the handicapped to limit their fertility. In the writings of the English neo-Malthusians there was also a strain of eugenic thinking based on the' fear that the better sort were in danger of being outbred by the inferior. Indeed, Francis Galton, the father of eugenics, and most of his closest followers were of the opinion that the main impact of birth control had been negative in nature inasmuch as it had been practiced mainly by those who owed it to the community to reproduce. The task posed modern society was to limit the breeding of the inferior and sponsor that of the superior. The neo-Malthusians argued, followed by Robin, that the best way to inhibit reproduction of inferior stock was by the dissemination of contraceptive information among the lower orders. Such eugenic arguments did not make much headway in France at the turn of the century, partly because the French were not as given to talk of racial stock as were the English and Germans. Georges Vacher de Lapouge, the antisemitic follower of Arthur de Gobineau, did discuss in *Les Sélections sociales* (1896) the relationship of racial purity to fertility and concluded that miscegenation was the root cause of France's low rate of natality, but his bizarre theories led to no practical policy recommendations.[25] More down to earth were the concerns expressed by Dr. Auguste Lutaud writing under the pseudonym "Dr. Minime" in 1891 in the *Journal de médecine de Paris* on "Le néo-Malthusianisme." Citing Bertillon's figures on the 1886 census of Paris, Lutaud pointed out that the wealthiest *quartiers* had the lowest birth rates and the poorest, the highest. The "degenerate" produced as a consequence a disproportionately high percentage of the next generation. In self-defense the nation would have to propagate among the poor methods of contraception while attempting to win the wealthy back to the traditionally large family.[26] This was the line that Robin was to follow in the 1890s as part of his initial campaign to win the support of the socially respectable. In 1896 he appealed in such terms to the Société d'anthropologie de Paris and later recapitulated his argument in a brochure entitled *Dégénérescence de l'espèce humaine: causes et remèdes*. The gist of his argument was that natural selection no longer effectively removed weak stock.[27] Thanks to advances in medicine and hygiene, those who might once have perished could now survive. If a better society were to be created, Robin asserted, the state could not support forever an increasing burden of misfits; the only sensible solution was to adopt a policy of what he referred to as "le méliorisme," by which the genetically weak would be provided with the means to avoid offspring through either contraception or sterilization.[28]

How Robin hoped to square his libertarian views with his eugenic concerns was never made clear, but two points raised by the issue must be stressed. First, Robin was far from being the only one on the left tantalized by the eugenic promise of improving the race. The eugenics message attracted mainly the "new" conservatives of the nineteenth century who saw in science a way of sustaining the status quo, but it also drew important numbers of reformers and revolutionaries imbued with the positivistic belief that no aspect of social life was immune to scientific improvement.[29] Second, Robin obviously hoped that his discussion of *le méliorisme* would act as bait to lure the respectable into publicly supporting birth control. He thus expressed his greatest interest in the topic in the early years of his campaign when he was assiduously attempting to win the attention of conservative organizations. In 1895 and 1896 he appealed to the Société d'anthropologie; in 1896 he produced a pamphlet *Aux Docteurs*, called on the Grand Orient Lodge of the Masons for support, and addressed the Congrès pour protéger et accroitre la population, and upon his return from New Zealand sent a note on overpopulation to the Humanitarian Congress meeting at the 1900 Paris Exhibition.[30] Once he determined that he was not going to receive the support of the established public leadership, Robin played down the eugenic side of his argument and accepted that the defense of birth control would remain of necessity primarily an issue of concern to libertarians.[31]

Robin's socialist-feminist interests provided the third and most important element in his birth control ideology. Here again it is possible to locate his thought in the context of the nineteenth-century French left. Although the leading socialists had exhibited a marked lack of sympathy for the discussion of fertility, Robin could turn to predecessors on the liberal and anarchistic fringes of the movement who would provide the first hesitant defenses of contraception. It has to be remembered that the nineteenth-century population debate was in part begun because Malthus was jolted into writing *An Essay on the Principles of Population* after detecting in the writings of A.N. de Condorcet (1743−94) an apparent sympathy for contraception. Referring to the Frenchman's prediction that in the future man would control his reproduction, Malthus declared:

> He then proceeds to remove the difficulty of overpopulation in a manner, which I profess not to understand. Having observed, that the ridiculous prejudices of superstition would by that time have ceased to throw over morals a corrupt and degrading austerity he alludes, either to a promiscuous concubinage, which would prevent breeding or to something else as unnatural. To remove the difficulty in this way, will, surely, in the opinion of most men, be, to destroy that virtue and purity of manners, which the advocates of equality, and of the perfectibility of man, profess to be the end and object of their views.[32]

Condorcet had in fact set the line of argument in his *Esquisse d'un tableau historique des progrès de l'esprit humain* (1794), which was to be followed by later birth control advocates. He wrote that soon

> ... men will then know that, if they have obligations to those beings
> who are not yet here, it consists not of bringing them into existence, but
> of making them happy; they have for their purpose the general
> well-being of the human species or of the society in which they live; of
> the family to which they are attached, and not the childish idea of
> burdening the world with useless and unfortunate beings.[33]

Condorcet had been one of the few philosophes to subject both the status
of women and the family to critical examination. He was not satisfied that
either had been predetermined by nature to continue in its present form,
and he thus had no qualms when it came to questioning the value of
population growth as a sign of public prosperity. The same question was
asked by Etienne de Sénacour (1770–1846) in De l'amour (1806):

> In Europe a quarter of the population cannot escape its abject poverty. It
> is true that this distress is not directly produced by the lack of space, and
> that foodstuffs are not wanting; but will the increasing of the population
> reform the habits that are to a large part a result of the number of men
> collected together under a single ruler?[34]

Condorcet and Sénacour did not suggest that population control would
solve every problem; they simply stated that the individual had a right to
contraception. More important, they were insisting that a woman had the
right to control her own body.

> The sex which forms and feeds has tasks to fulfill; often it wishes to avoid
> them, often it even must. It is the sex which receives the action which has
> the right of refusing it. . . . Men finding no danger here for themselves
> easily forget what harm is done in making pregnant a woman who
> cannot want it. They cannot ignore how odious such indifference is, and
> all that there is contemptible in this brutal abandonment. But what they
> almost all seem to ignore is that even in the unions sanctioned by the
> law, it is imprudent, blameworthy, senseless, to have as many children
> as chance in some way produces.[35]

Condorcet and Sénancour accepted the notion that pleasure was an
obvious measure of happiness and that women had as much right to
pleasure as men.[36] In contrast to those who called for the repression of the
passions, they optimistically held that, once freed of the trammels of family
and society, the free expression of human needs could only lead to good.

The most famous defender of such liberty in the nineteenth century
was Charles Fourier (1772–1837). The artificial restriction of fertility was
in his eyes a natural enough practice. "The father and the mother
frequently seek by artifice to prevent . . . birth,"[37] he wrote, and he

castigated the priests who censured "certain precautions that prudence dictates. *Interdicto semen effundendi extra va debitum* [It is prohibited to produce semen except to fulfill one's proper duty]." He seemed to believe, however, that such practices would not have to be pursued forever, because the very freedom of the passions in his "état sociétaire" would ensure a stable population. He was attacked for promulgating contraceptive theories, but in fact he was hopelessly utopian when it came to the problem of assuring a low birth rate.[38] He believed that women would become less prolific due to greater activity, a "régime gastrosophique," "moeurs phanérogames," and "exercise intégral."[39] Moreover, he declared that the changes he envisaged would not come into force until at least a generation after the founding of harmony.[40] Contemporaries were not taken in by these reservations. They recognized that Fourier was clearly advancing a line of thought that defended the right of birth control. He was a resolute critic of the family that served to oppress both the woman and the child. He was a feminist but his feminism, unlike that of his contemporaries, did not consist of seeking to restrict men to the chaste condition heretofore demanded of women. Instead of calling for the mortification of the flesh and the holding in check of sexual feelings, he gloried in their free expression.[41]

By his defense of women's right to work in the meetings of the International and by his practical efforts to promote coeducation at Cempuis, Robin had already given abundant proof of his concern for women's rights. In his birth control campaign activities he sought to complement the Fourierist stress on the freedom of the woman with the provision of contraceptive information, which might make such freedoms a reality. His first step in this direction was the establishment of a dispensary in Paris in 1889 from which handbills were distributed that proclaimed:

> Mothers of families, young women who soon will be, all you who wish to assure yourselves of a lasting happiness, learn what every woman should know, consult Mmes L . . . and Co., teachers of hygiene, whose wise opinions are based on the most certain data of the science of life and society. You will bless for the rest of your life the day of your visit.[42]

In 1895 he followed up this appeal with a series of handbills including *Aux gens mariés!* and *Femmes, soeurs bien-aimées*. The key passage of the former read:

> The greatest comfort that one can give to an anxious wife is to indicate to her safe, effective means of becoming a mother only when she has after careful reflection decided to do so. *It is the first step, the essential point of the real emancipation of woman*, and in turn of the entire race.[43]

And in the latter pamphlet Robin counseled women on their right to control their fertility.

> This depends on you, you are absolutely the mistresses of your destiny. It is necessary that you do not ignore the fact, neither you nor your companions in suffering, that *science has emancipated you from the frightening fate of being mothers against your will.* [44]

Robin did not always see eye-to-eye with orthodox feminists, but he placed the rights of women at the center of his defense of birth control. The first number of *Régénération* in 1896 declared the Ligue's goal to be to "win for woman the FREEDOM of MATERNITY."[45] This freedom Robin saw as restricted in the first instance by the teachings of the church that sought to inculcate in women's minds real and imaginary terrors. Even after marriage the woman could find herself subjected to the unfeeling demands of a husband in a relationship that was little better than prostitution.[46] Sexual intercourse, Robin asserted, was an essential ingredient of a healthy life but could only be fully appreciated by the woman freed from religious prejudices by a scientific education and freed from fear of pregnancy by knowledge of birth control.[47]

It was to the socialist and anarchist left that Robin turned as the natural defenders of such rights. Birth control, he claimed, had to be viewed as a tactic worthy of their interest because of the attacks made on it by priests, generals, capitalists, chauvinists — all the "procréatomanes."[48] The upper classes, as every one knew, employed contraceptives themselves but through shameless hypocrisy were using appeals to morality, decency, and national need to prevent their being obtained by those who most needed them. In addition Robin held out the hope that fertility control could play some role in strengthening labor by restricting the employer's access to large number of workers; the birth strike or "grève de ventre" could be made part of the tactic of the general strike.[49] And lastly Robin warned that since the victory of birth control was inevitable, it would be to the left's discredit if it were not numbered among its supporters.

> It would be a pity for the history of official socialism that it [the victory] occurred *despite* it. It is already bad enough that our successes until now have been obtained *without* its support.[50]

Until 1896 birth control had been discussed positively in France only in one public lecture by Mme. Huot and in a medical brochure published anonymously by Dr. Lutaud. From the turn of the century until 1908 Robin's indefatigable efforts made the subject a topic of national debate. The message carried in *Régénération* was more or less an elaboration of Robin's views on Malthusian economics, eugenics, feminism, and socialism. The Ligue's main concerns were to win as many influential recruits as possible and to provide practical contraceptive information to the masses. By 1900 when an international meeting of neo-Malthusians was held in Paris, the Ligue could count as supporters not only J.B. Clément, Eugène Fournière, and Adrien Meslier but also Dr. Lapique of the Sorbonne, Dr. Alfred Naquet, the influential socialist and "father of French divorce," and Charles Malato, editor of *L'Aurore*.[51] *Régénération* appeared monthly carrying reports of Robin's lectures, which were usually held in bourses du travail, the local union halls. In his work he was assisted by new recruits: his son-in-law Gabriel Giroud, the feminist Nelly Roussel, and, most important of all, the young anarchist Eugène Humbert.[52] To avoid prosecution under the law against "les associations philosophiques," the Ligue proper consisted of less than twenty persons associated for the purposes of publishing the journal. Such precautions were necessary. Those associated with the Ligue's activities were, because of their involvement with anarchists, subject to police surveillance and occasional prosecution. In 1900 the secretary-treasurer of the Ligue was fined for distributing a birth control tract; in 1901 Sicard-Palange was prosecuted in Bordeaux for selling Robin's *Santé de la femme*; in 1904 the *Réveil syndical* of Lens was similarly tried for printing a neo-Malthusian article; in 1906 a certain Émile Hamelin who was distributing both antimilitarist and Ligue material was arrested in Trelazé; in 1907 Victor Cornil, the Ligue representative in Roubaix, was prosecuted, and in 1908 Dr. Fernand Elosu, another anarchist-pacifist, was jailed for two months in Bayonne for selling *L'Amour inféconde*.[53]

Typical of the Ligue's propagandizing efforts was the discussion of birth control held at a meeting of the Union syndical du bronze at the Paris Bourse du travail on June 23, 1903.[54] The speakers included Charles Desplanques, Auguste Liard-Courtois, "Libertad" (Joseph Albert, the founder of *L'Anarchie*), V.J. Gelez, and Mme. Louise Reville. It was in the ranks of the syndicalists that the Ligue found its most active supporters, but the working-class audience was more interested in practical information than in abstract theorizing. When the speakers drifted too far afield, they were interrupted by cries of "Les moyens!" To respond to such demands the Ligue sold tracts such as *Aux femmes, Aux gens mariés*, and *Moyens d'éviter les grands familles* for fifty centimes, Allbutt's *Le livre de l'épouse* for one franc, and Drysdale's *Eléments de science sociale* for three francs fifty.[55] Detailed information was also provided on how douching was to be carried out, how primitive condoms could be made from animal intestines, and how soluble pessaries could be prepared at home. Concerning the latter, Robin provided a recipe for a "pâté préservative" consisting of gelatine, glycerine, and quinine, a mixture which he insisted produced a product as reliable as the commercial brands of pessaries.[56] It was, however, by the sale of contraceptives that the Ligue made much of its income. Ads were carried in *Régénération* for a variety of condoms, both the soluble and Mensinga pessaries, douches, douching solutions, and bidets. And finally, for those who sought personal information the journal declared that consultations were offered by medical practitioners whose addresses would be provided on demand.[57]

By the turn of the century the commercial opportunities offered by the sale of birth control material was such that businessmen with no ideological interest in population control began to enter the market. In Doctor Brennus's *Amour et securité*, which first appeared in 1893 and boasted 108 editions by 1906, there were advertisements for pessaries ("ovule antiseptique") douches, sponges, bidets, contraceptive powders ("Le Philutérus"), diaphragms ("fosset utérophite"), vaginal protectors ("L'Infaillible"), *capuchons* ("Bonnet fin-de-siècle"), *baudruches*, condoms in a variety of colors and imitation crocodile hide, as well as a list of "novelties" including "ceintures électrique," "pommades virginale," "anneaus contre la spermathorrhée," "ceintures de chasteté," and "serviettes pour menses."[58] The Ligue de la régénération humaine was far from being the sole purveyor of contraceptives, but it did have a source of income from which to finance its propaganda activities. By 1908 disagreements over the employment of the funds (which were in a state of confusion as a result of Robin's anarchistic disregard for the niceties of bookkeeping) as well as the desire of some younger men to throw off the heavy-handed leadership of the old libertarian, led to the breakup of the Ligue.[59] Robin withdrew from active campaigning, and *Régénération* disappeared to be replaced by two competing journals, *Le Malthusien* and *Génération consciente*. The former paper under the editorship of Albert Gros began its life carrying attacks against the dictatorial policies of Robin and went so far as to cast aspersions on his morality.[60] Gros and his followers formed the Ligue néo-malthusienne de France, which was marked by a greater degree of individualism than the old league. Cautiously avoiding political involvements and (at least until 1911) even relationships with other birth control groups, the writers of *Le Malthusien* were spared police repression. The new paper's defense of birth control was not all that different from Robin's except for a more pronounced interest in eugenics. It cited the growth of interest in the science in England, warmly reviewed Tarbouriech's book which touched on the subject, and hailed the 1912 London Eugenics Conference as providing birth control with a new respectability.[61] The paper's skirting of confrontations with authority and its lack of interest in the socialist cause gave it a more conservative tenor. It did attract, however, some important contributors of the individualist-anarchist stripe such as Manuel Devaldès and Emile Armand, who would both play an important role in advancing the cause of sex radicalism in France. Nor did the paper's caution prevent it from treating the opponents of birth control with caustic disdain. In its columns all pronatalist policies were referred to as "projets lapinistes," the leading populationist Senator René Béranger labeled "Père La Pudeur," and a conference on vice called "le congrès des pornomanes."[62] Indeed, in its enthusiasm to ridicule the enemies of neo-Malthusianism, the *Malthusien* was by 1912 supporting its erstwhile rival *Génération consciente*.

Génération consciente under the editorship of Eugène Humbert from 1908 to 1914 followed, if anything, a more politically engaged line of argument than *Régénération* had in defense of birth control. Humbert came from the working class, the illegitimate child of an officer and a working woman.[63] Apprenticed to a cobbler, he was drawn to the anarchism espoused by Jean Grave's movement known as *Liberté*. Through the libertarian educational experiments of the Université populaire he met Paul Robin, who won him to the cause of fertility control. Humbert in turn was successful in recruiting other anarchists to the cause, Sebastian Faure being the best known. In the first number of *Génération consciente* which appeared on April 15, 1908, Humbert spelled out his reasons for the necessity of the rational control of fertility. First came its importance to women.

> In teaching woman the ways in which to avoid conception when she does not desire it, we put an end to the disadvantageous state in which nature placed her vis-à-vis man and which society has so odiously abused; we prepare her emancipation.[64]

Second, birth control could assure a better fate for children; third, it guaranteed immediate benefits to the working class as a whole, while in no way replacing the need for social change. What was not mentioned by Humbert was the Malthusian fear of overpopulation and this omission was matched by his journal's explicit denunciation of eugenics.[65] The contributor Auguste Liard-Courtois, for example, who had been a prison inmate himself, declared that thieves were not born but were created by their environment.[66]

The self-consciously radical tone of *Génération consciente* was not restricted to simple questions of fertility. It made a point of parading its antimilitarist sympathies and its anticlericalism. Priests were referred to as *les tondus*, and their injunctions against contraception met with crude banter. "God blesses large families, it's true," wrote one contributor "but he only had one son."[67] Because of the paper's close anarchist ties and the goading of René Béranger's Fédération des sociétés contre la pornographie, Humbert's group found itself under police surveillance. In 1909 after addressing an audience of over eight hundred in Rouen, both Humbert and Liard-Courtois were arrested and jailed for two months; in 1912 a certain Cauvin was fined three hundred francs in Marseilles for distributing neo-Malthusian tracts; in December of the same year Humbert was sentenced to another six months in prison for his activities; and in January of 1913 Dr. Liptay was fined for the same offense.[68] Strictly speaking, the prosecutions were not against the defense of birth control; there was no law making such an act a crime. Rather, the authorities bent the laws on abortion and those against outrages to morals in an attempt to silence the propagandists.

The persecution of Humbert and his troop only drove them on. By 1910 they claimed to have distributed over 120,000 handbills and 10,000 catalogues while selling 125,000 copies of Gabriel Giroud's *Moyens d'éviter la grossesse* and 140,000 of Jean Marestan's *L'Education sexuelle*.[69] Original forms of propaganda included a column in *Génération consciente* entitled "The Example Comes From Above," in which the number of children had by leading deputies was listed — for example, Viviani — 0, Doumergue — 0, Trouillot — 2, Millerand — 1 — and cartoons such as that which appeared in June 1912 entitled "L'Affranchi," which depicted a woman crying, "Mon ventre, c'est a moi . . . seule!" while facing down the representatives of the church, business, and the military.[70] The most dramatic forms of campaigning remained the public lectures in the provinces, which provided occasions for distributing tracts, winning the attention of local radical publications, and precipitating confrontations with pronatalist forces. In 1913 over a hundred such meetings were addressed by Humbert, and new militants joined the fray including Louis Grandidier, secretary of the Bourse du travail of St. Denis, Eugène Lericolais, editor of the *Socialiste de l'Ouest*, Léon Marinot, a leading member of the Chevalier du travail, and André Lorulot and Franc Sutor, both active anarchists. Perhaps the most striking aspect of the campaign led by the team of *Génération consciente* was its concern to make information concerning contraception and sexuality in general as accessible as possible to the working class. The paper carried clear accounts accompanied by illustrations on the employment of douches, pessaries, and other contraceptive devices. Dr. Fernand Mascaux of Brussels also contributed a column in which he lectured the readership on everything from the necessity of a woman employing a "serviette" during her period to the ways in which to deal with masturbation.[71] Like its sister papers, *Génération consciente* also advertised commercial contraceptives like "Le Perfect" and "L'Imperméable," from the sale of which it financed its activities. The arrangement was not only monetarily rewarding; it complemented the anarchists' desire to win a degree of self-sufficiency for the workers.[72] The fact that the English Malthusian League did not provide such services was commented on by Giroud in 1910. "The English propagandist leaves the responsibility of the diffusion of neo-Malthusian appliances to merchants."[73] The French activists saw themselves as playing some part in overthrowing the existing economic system whereas their English counterparts had no such desires.

By the outbreak of World War I France had, in large part due to the activities of Paul Robin, an active birth control movement that challenged both the left and the right to declare themselves on the issue of fertility. That the campaign for fertility control — despite the disclaimers of the leading socialists and anarchists — was indelibly marked by Robin's leftist origins was to be the crucial factor in determining the particular types of recruits drawn to the cause, to be discussed in chapter seven.

CHAPTER SEVEN

Political and Sexual Radicalism

Where did the support for Paul Robin's propagandizing activities originate? It did not come from the ranks of the leading socialists. The spokesmen for the socialist parties continued to oppose the public discussion of the artificial restriction of family size. In England, where the Malthusian League combined pleas for population control with socially conservative economic pronouncements, labor's suspicion of such a movement appeared to be well warranted. In France, however, the birth control campaign was led by men of the left. Indeed, English Malthusians were somewhat taken aback by the revolutionary views of Robin and his followers. Very little was said in the *Malthusian* about the socialistic and anarchistic aspects of the French group, but once the continental movement was crushed by government legislation, the English asserted that such a fate had been the price necessarily paid for its "anticapitalistic and revolutionary views."[1] Given the socially advanced views of Robin, why did he have so little success in winning the support of the most prominent leftist politicians? They, of course, in the main, were repeating the arguments expressed by the socialists of the first half of the nineteenth century who, as we have seen, equated a defense of fertility control with social conservatism. What was new about the situation in the late 1890s, however, was the fact that Paul Robin, a well-known libertarian, was leading the birth control campaign while the most vociferous populationists were on the right. The leaders of the left accordingly found the discussion of fertility an embarrassment. No socialist of the latter half of the nineteenth century would rival the misogyny of Proudhon, but most remained rigidly conservative when analyzing the family. At the September 1867 meeting of the International Working Men's Association, Robin was incited by the expression of such views to make one of his first statements on the need to reexamine traditional sex roles. Cesar de Paepe of Belgium read the majority report of the International's commission on women's work, which consisted primarily of a denigration of female labor outside the home as "unnatural."

> Following the laws of nature it is therefore necessary to consider every woman as destined to become a wife and consequently a homemaker,

110

then mother, and accordingly charged with the education and instruction of her children, and if today all do not fulfill this destiny it is necessary to blame social prejudices which lead to unfortunate marriages, and poverty, the mother of prostitution, and the progress of Malthusian mores; in a word it is necessary to hold responsible the existing social order.[2]

Robin responded by writing with Hins and Eslens the minority report attacking de Paepe's implicit denial of the woman's right to lead an independent life.[3] It would be this concern for the rights of the individual which led Robin, after leaving the International, to devote himself to the propagation of just those Malthusian mores that de Paepe had castigated.

In Germany some socialist leaders did take the population question seriously. Karl Kautsky showed some interest in contraception in *Der Einfluss der Volkersvermehrung* (1888), as did August Bebel in *Die Frau und der Sozialismus* (1883).[4] In Russia even Lenin grudgingly admitted in 1913, "The freedom of medical propaganda and the defense of the elementary democratic rights of male and female citizens is one thing. The social theory of neo-Malthusianism is another."[5] In France few took the effort to make such a distinction. No leader of any stature among the French socialists took a stand on the issue. The "scientific socialists" avoided most of the pious moralizing of the earlier utopians while skirting the question of woman's right to avoid pregnancy. It would appear that in the face of the wide-scale family planning from the 1870s on, socialists felt it was prudent to avoid the issue. Jean Jaurès gave no clear responses to demands for his opinions on the subject; Léon Blum implied in *Du mariage* (1907) that contraception was necessary but he kept his thoughts cloaked in hazy verbiage.[6]

Actual critiques of Robin's activities were left to lesser lights. The first response made by socialists to the creation of Robin's Ligue was an article by Desiré Descamps in the *Revue socialiste* of 1897. In the previous year Descamps had already broached the population issue in an essay in which he attributed the fall of fertility to capitalism.[7] Industrial society imposed sterility on women by depriving them of the roles of wife and mother. The view that capitalism was the main cause of the population problem was to be the key argument of succeeding generations of socialist critics. For Descamps the entry of Robin — this "disciple hétérodox de Malthus" — into the fray was simply a sign of his ignorance of the nature of basic economic and political oppression. Godwin, Leroux, Proudhon, Guesde, Valette, and Bonnier had all recognized the antisocial nature of Malthus's message, but Descamps concluded that this verity had escaped Robin, as had the evidence that contraception employed by the healthier classes threatened France with national degeneration.[8]

The linking of capitalism and depopulation was continued by Dr. Pax Salvat in *La dépopulation de la France* (1903), in which he asserted that working women were being prevented from having children by their need to work, middle-class women by their lack of maternal feeling. Capitalism had thus produced what Salvat pejoratively labeled as a "feminisme inférieure" of the workers and a "feminisme supérieure" of the idle.[9]

In a more thoughtful contribution to the fertility debate, Henri Dagan in "Réponse aux néo-Malthusiens" (1903) suggested that Robin and his ilk were blind to the fact that capitalists wanted the workers to have smaller families. Dagan conceded that deputies — "Most of these old gentlemen who have not stopped tricking nature, be it with their mistresses, be it with their wives" — liked to pose as defenders of the large family while hypocritically limiting the size of their own.[10] He also accepted the fact that conservative papers such as *Temps, Peuple française, Echo de Paris,* and *Figaro* featured populationists' editorials. But Dagan went on to assert that Robin was on the wrong track because first, the contraceptive means Robin suggested — "le petit arsenal d'instruments" — could not be employed by the masses because they were ineffective, inapplicable, dangerous, and too expensive; second, even if birth control by the workers were possible, it could not serve as a universal panacea; and third, Malthusian economics were faulty in that it was underconsumption, not overpopulation, that was the cause of poverty.[11] The most interesting point made by Dagan was that despite all the talk of a "birth strike," business was not concerned by declining fertility and might actually desire it. In a prophetic passage that foresaw the Rockefellers' active support for birth control research later in the century Dagan declared,

> One could even foresee, without any great effort at divination, the formation of some powerful oligarchy of which the Carnegie, Rockeffeler [sic], Pierpont-Morgan millionaires are the precursors, an all-powerful oligarchy. . . . It would no longer need a prolific people. On the contrary, they could pose a danger to it. All it would have to have under its control would be a small but well-trained proletariat, a servant and accessory of the perfected mechanism that would be sufficient to assure an abundant and varied production.[12]

In passing, Dagan also rejected Robin's assertion that birth control could lead to the revitalizing of the working class. In 1907 Dr. Oguse expressed the same thoughts in declaring his sorrow that some on the left were attracted to neo-Malthusianism by the seductive, though erroneous, view that simply the provision of contraceptive pamphlets would result in the "regeneration" of mankind. Such a social heresy had to be based on the premise that population could be manipulated regardless of the social system. In fact, Oguse argued, capitalism necessarily elicited a certain type of population growth. In such a system labor could never be "free" either to procreate or to refrain from doing so. To suggest that it could was to imply that a means of avoiding the class struggle existed. For these reasons Oguse did not find it surprising that those opposed to the Revolution — he referred to them as "des gens considérables" — would back the birth control campaign. What about working-class couples who sought short-term gains by limiting their family size? They were, said Oguse, equivalent to counterfeiters whose prosperity damaged that of the community.[13]

Such attacks on couples who "betrayed" the labor movement were not unique. Dr. Vargas was even more strident:

> We do not want a happier proletariat, working families better dressed, living more hygienically, children shielded from dangerous *promiscuities*, working-class women no longer exposed to the dangers of repeated abortions: we want the suppression of the proletariat, even the possibility of an unhygienic existence for certain families; we want the atrocious dilemma "Either do not procreate or expose your children to hunger, misery, and illness" to no longer even be posed. And every theory that proposes improvements in the existing state of things we wish to suppress and not improve warrants only our hostility.[14]

Robert Hertz's pamphlet *Socialisme et dépopulation* (1910) contained the same sort of argument.

> Of course if it pleases a proletarian family to improve its situation in having no children, they are free to do so: it is a personal affair which is their business. But in remaining sterile, they have no more contributed to the emancipation of their class than a worker who becomes a wine merchant has abolished wage-earning.[15]

If the working class as a whole adopted such practices, the result would be an "amoindrissement national," a rise in unemployment as the number of consumers fell, and a decline of the socialist population relative to the hoards of prolific "barbares," i.e., Catholics and foreign laborers. The working-class family which had only one child would not produce a socialist militant; "il fera le plus souvent un petit bourgeois bien sage ou un arriviste médiocre." Like many of his socialist colleagues, Hertz concluded by taking the somewhat contradictory position of condemning the neo-Malthusians for their actions while simultaneously asserting that they had no real success.

> As for the neo-Malthusians, it is to give them too much credit to attribute to their propaganda an important role in such a general state of affairs; they have only provided an economic justification, which is in any event

erroneous, for one of the profound and irresistible tendencies of our time.[16]

Hertz's pamphlet was warmly received in *Revue socialiste*.[17] In light of this support, as well as Guesde's and Lafargue's hostility to Robin's campaign, and Jaurès's and Vaillant's silence, it became abundantly clear that birth control was not to receive the official support of the socialists.[18]

The leading anarchists were just as distant. Their opposition to Robin's crusade was based first on their belief that neo-Malthusianism began with a pessimistic assessment of man's potential, and second, on their traditional views of the sex roles. Robin had, as a result of his involvement in the International, long friendships with Guillaume, Reclus, Grave, and Kropotkin, but these relationships were all marred by clashes over the population issue. At the bottom of James Guillaume's opposition was a marked antipathy toward feminism. In September 1866 he declared:

> The family is the foundation of society; the place of the woman is at the domestic hearth; we not only oppose her abandoning it to sit in a political assembly or to operate a club, we do not even wish, were it possible, for her to leave it to undertake industrial work.[19]

Inspired by such sentiments, Guillaume, along with Peter Kropotkin, successfully opposed Robin's attempts at the Saint Imier conference of 1877 to have the anarchists take up the discussion of fertility control. In 1905 he went so far as to accuse Robin, by his launching of the Ligue de la régénération humaine, of being guilty of "ridiculing the cause of the emancipation of labor which you claim to serve."[20] Kropotkin was a close friend of Robin during their exile in London in the 1870s but strangely enough does not mention him once in his *Autobiography*. No doubt this omission was due to the acrimony that grew as a result of their differing views on population and the family. Kropotkin supported Guillaume, as we have seen, and likewise informed Robin, "You are holding back the revolution."[21] The basis of Kropotkin's anger was his rather vague, romantic views of women and his optimistic belief in the infinite potential of a rationally administered world, delineated in works such as *Fields, Factories, and Workshops* (1899). Jean Grave presented similar utopian views in *La société future* (1895) while he ridiculed the pessimistic fears of Malthusians. He assumed, as did many on the left, that eventually the development of civilization would act as a force to naturally lower fecundity. In the short term he declared that fear of pregnancy itself served as a moderating influence on population growth. "For the rest, the sufferings of childbirth, the inconveniences of pregnancy, will still be in place to provide a moderating control on proliferation."[22] Such an assertion revealed his lack of empathy for women faced with undesired pregnancies as did his sneering reference to Robin's concern for birth control as "un dada." Equal in stature to Grave on the French anarchist left and equally opposed to Robin was Elisée Reclus. In his *L'Evolution, la révolution, et l'idéal anarchique* (1898) appeared the mandatory, optimistic appraisal of nature's bounty; the spread of Malthusian doctrines Reclus attributed to the hard-hearted bourgeoisie. In *Union libres* (1899) Reclus did defend a more open form of marriage, but as Robin himself pointed out, love could hardly be called "free" if the woman remained subjected to unwanted conceptions.[23] Nevertheless, even the leading woman anarchist, Madeleine Vernet, declared her opposition to Robin's campaign in *Le Libertaire*.[24]

The most prominent leaders of the French left refused to lend their support to Robin's campaign, but their pronouncements did not do full justice to the widespread interest taken by radicals in the question of sexuality during the Belle Epoque. Victor Serge recalled in his *Memoirs of a Revolutionary* that before the First World War the libertarian subculture of France and Belgium was preoccupied by the relationship of sex to politics. The same links were forged elsewhere in Europe. In Spain the anarchist educator Francesco Ferrer served as conduit for Robin's theories, in England Henry Seymour declared in *The Anarchy of Love* (1888) that contraception was indispensable for sexual freedom, in Italy even Benito Mussolini lent his support, while on his passage from syndicalism to fascism, to Dr. Luigi Berta, the founder of an Italian neo-Malthusian League.[25]

Who in France supported Robin's *Régénération* and later Humbert's *Génération consciente*? Adherents primarily came from the margins of the political world. First among them would be anticlericals drawn to a campaign that promised to undermine the powers of religion. Robin was the president of the French section of the International Association of Freethinkers and could accordingly count on the help of many of those of similar persuasion.[26] In addition he was a Mason. Jean Bidegrain claimed in *Le grand orient de France* (1905) that as a consequence the Masonic Lodges defended Robin for his educational experiments at Cempuis in the 1880s and later provided a forum in which Dr. Adrien Meslier publicized his birth control activities.[27]

Mention of Dr. Meslier brings one to yet another semisecret organization in which Robin had allies, the Chevalerie du travail français. The Chevalerie, inspired by the American Knights of Labor, was the last of the French nineteenth-century clandestine artisanal organizations. From its ranks came Dr. Meslier, an active militant of the Parti ouvrier in Clichy and Saint Ouen. Meslier's intimate knowledge of poverty and illness gained by

116   SEXUALITY AND SOCIAL ORDER

his experiences as a slum doctor led him to support the birth control
campaign. Elected deputy, he, along with Victor Dejeante and Anatole
Sixte-Quenin, were the only representatives to defend neo-Malthusian
doctrines in the Assembly. In addition the Chevalerie included Léon
Marinot, a self-educated worker and labor organizer in the nineteenth
arrondissement, who with Meslier in 1898 gave one of the first public
defenses of Robin's creed at the Maison du peuple on the rue Ramey;
André Levy-Oulman, a Mason and barrister known for his defense of
antimilitarists, who in 1911 was the only lawyer to sign an open letter to
Senator René Béranger protesting the persecutions of birth controllers;
Octave Martinet, an old Blanquist and friend of Robin's who ran a
pharmacie on the rue Geoffrey Saint-Hilaire from which propaganda was
diffused; and Jean Colly, a miner's son whose positions as municipal
councilor for the Bercy *quartier* and eventually deputy for the Seine
permitted him to provide the neo-Malthusians with a degree of support.[28]

Other deputies sympathetic to the battles waged by *Régénération*
included Victor Dejeante, an active anticlerical and antimilitarist who rose
from humble origins to become deputy for Belleville; Eugène Fournière,
deputy for the Aisne and one-time editor of *Revue socialiste* who joined
Robin's Ligue in 1898; and Anatole Sixte-Quenin, a blacksmith's son from
Arles who as deputy from 1910 to the 1930s combined an interest in sex
reform with anticolonialism, anticlericalism, and antimilitarism. The best
known of all the deputies to broach the subject of birth control, however,
was Alfred Naquet. Of Jewish heritage but raised as a freethinker, Naquet
began political life a Blanquist, passed his middle years a Boulangist, and
ended up a socialist. His concern with moral questions and his long
campaign for the reintroduction of the legalization of the dissolution of
marriage earned him the title "père de divorce." Naquet's critical analysis
of marriage in *Religion, propriété, famille* (1896), *Temps futurs* (1900),
and *L'Humanité et la patrie* (1901) predisposed him to accept the
importance of the issue of family planning. He was careful, however, to
subject the doctrines of the birth controllers themselves to careful scrutiny
and in *Néo-Malthusianisme et socialisme* (1910) made it clear that though
the control of conception was obviously essential it was an error to assume
that birth control by itself could produce a better society.[29]

The activities of Meslier, Dejeante, Fournière, Sixte-Quenin, and
Naquet provides evidence that birth control was not without support even
within the socialist camp. More dramatic proof was offered by the
placarding of the department of Basses-Pyrénées in April 1911 with a
proabortion poster purportedly of socialist origins. It read:

> The socialist party publicly declares the following principles . . . A
> woman should have the right of ending an undesired pregnancy in

having herself aborted with the legal aid of a doctor; abortion carried out
in this fashion and at an early date, freed of all quackery, would mean
that no longer would the woman run the risks of an operation carried out
secretly by the inexperienced and the incompetent; abortion would thus
become a normal operation posing no risks. The act of voluntary
abortion would therefore constitute neither a crime nor misdemeanor,
for neither the woman nor the abortionist.[30]

The authors of the declaration refused to identify themselves, however,
and party officials denied all responsibility. For such outspoken defenses of
sexual freedom one had to turn to ranks of the libertarians.

Eugène Humbert was, as we have seen, first drawn to active political
engagement via the anarchists, and he in turn succeeded in leading many
libertarians to accept the defense of birth control as logically necessary in
any defense of individual rights. The most important of his converts was
Sébastien Faure. An anti-Malthusian, as he made clear in early works such
as *La douleur universelle* (1895), Faure by 1903 had taken up the cause of
fertility control on the grounds that it could provide a more healthy,
intelligent youth who would prepare the way for the Revolution. Faure also
saw the need for libertarians to embrace the birth control campaign and
thus strike a blow against the traditionally male-dominated, authoritarian
family structure.[31] It was the potentially subversive nature of contraception
that similarly attracted the following: the anarchist theoretician Charles
Malato; Henri Gauche who wrote as René Chaugi in *Temps nouveaux*;
the Dreyfusard and antimilitarist Degoulet who contributed to *Génération
consciente* under the name of Urbain Gohier; the pacifist Joseph Albert
known as "Libertad"; André Roulot who, under the name of André
Lorulot, published *Anarchie* with "Libertad" and in 1910 wrote
Procréation consciente; Clément Janin, the editor of *Action*; the anarchist
and ex-convict Auguste Liard-Courtois; and the Belgian libertarian Victor
Dave who introduced both Emma Goldman and Margaret Sanger to the
Parisian world of sex radicals.[32]

Sharing many of the political views of the anarchists was a second
group of adherents who were, however, preoccupied more with the
question of sex reform than with politics. The most important was Robin's
son-in-law Gabriel Giroud, who in addition to writing the former's
biography, produced a number of birth control tracts before the war under
the noms de guerre of G. Hardy and C. Lyon. It was his contention that
birth control had "consequences feministes" inasmuch as it allowed
women access to public life; this concern for women's rights led him from
defending contraception to accepting the necessity of abortion. He
criticized socialists such as Guesde and Jaurès for failing to support Robin
as well as eugenists such as Forel and Wylm for ignoring the role

contraception could play in improvement of national vigor.[33] Writers who followed Giroud's lead included Henri Coudon, who under the name Victor Méric, produced Le problème sexuel (1910), and Gaston Harvard, who under the name of Jean Marestan, produced L'education sexuelle (1910). In the interwar period Giroud represented the French neo-Malthusians at international birth control conferences, while at home his efforts were supported by a second generation of sex radicals. Perhaps the most remarkable was Ernest Jouin, who wrote under the name of Emile Armand. He began his public life as a recruit of the Salvation Army but left both it and his wife when at the turn of the century he founded "L'ère nouvelle," a Christian anarchist group reminiscent of Tolstoy's movement. Armand's prewar publications supporting contraception included De la liberté sexuelle (1906), Le Malthusianisme, le néo-Malthusianisme, et le point de vue de l'individualisme (1910), and La Procréation volontaire (1912).[34] A contemporary of Armand was Ernest-Edmond Lohy, who wrote under the name of Manuel Devaldès. What drew Devaldès to Génération consciente — as he made clear in tracts such as La Chair à canon (1908) and La Brute prolifique (1914) — was the belief that overpopulation led to war and therefore birth control naturally complemented other antimilitarist campaigns.[35]

A source of tension in many of the short-lived pamphlet works supporting birth control resulted from their authors' espousing both anarchist and eugenic dogmas. As seen earlier Robin himself never fully squared his libertarianism with his belief that the race could be in some way regenerated by control of conceptions. The same double-edged message was carried in the works of Jean Marestan, Gabriel Giroud, Manuel Devaldès, and André Lorulot.[36] Ernest Tarbouriech, the expert in work safety legislation, though he praised Robin for being the first French writer to raise the importance of controlling fertility, reveled in the authoritarian ends to which such power could be turned if wielded by the state. In La Cité future: essai d'une utopie scientifique (1902) he sketched out the picture of a society in which government would sterilize the unfit, medically examine those about to marry, oblige mothers to have hospital births and nurse their young, and finally practice euthanasia on the decrepit.[37] Thus there was in Robin's stress on the greater efficiency offered by the rational planning of pregnancies a theme which could attract some support outside the libertarian camp.

Anarchist critics and journalists who enlisted in the struggle for birth control found their efforts paralleled by many writers and artists motivated not so much by schemes for political reform or sex education as by a basic sympathy for women subjected to unwanted pregnancies. Their numbers included Octave Mirbeau, anarchist sympathizer and anticlerical, the old

Communard poet J.B. Clément, who joined the Ligue in 1898, the syndicalist poet Eugène Lericolais, author of *Peu d'enfants: Pourquoi: Comment* (1912), Laurent Tailhade, who provided a preface for Lericolais's pamphlet but was best known for his defense of Vaillant's bomb attack on the Assembly with the words, "Qu'importe les victimes si le geste est beau?", and the symbolist poet Remy de Gourmont, who was one of the first to rally to Robin's defense in 1897 and respond to Béranger's purity campaign in 1906 with the assertion that the senator's ideal marriage was one in which there was "the minimum of contact and, during the operation some psalm or refrigerating prayer recited."[38]

The anarchist publications for which these writers wrote at the turn of the century are perhaps best known today not for the articles they printed but for the illustrations they carried by such graphic masters as Théophile Steinlin and Félix Vallotton. Some included explicit defenses of birth control. *Le Canard sauvage* dedicated a special issue of 5 July 1903 to the subject of "Repopulation." Steinlin contributed a cartoon of one working-class woman saying to another: "Have children! If we weren't dumb animals we'd leave that job to the rich"; while Roubille's picture of the bodies of dead soldiers was accompanied by the sardonic caption "It's for this that it's necessary to have boys."[39] Between 1902 and 1907 *L'Assiette au beurre* printed similar illustrations on the topics of abortion and clerical interference.[40]

Of all the artistic defenses of fertility control, however, the most interesting was a series of plays and novels clearly colored by neo-Malthusian preoccupations. Eugenic considerations occupied a central place in André Couvreur's novel *La famille: la graine* (1903), in which the lack of attention paid to the crucial question of conception was shown to be responsible for the spread of alcoholism, tuberculosis, and syphilis. Michel Corday's *Sesame ou la maternité consentie* (1903) was a plea for the discovery of better forms of contraception. The plot revolved around the fact that a man whose father has discovered an elixir that controls conceptions believes at first such a discovery could only serve the egotistical and ambitious but in the end sees that it alone will allow for women's full emancipation. In Brieux's famous play *Maternité* (1903) a similar argument was made, that only by way of better contraception could abortions and suicides brought on by seduction be avoided. Even in a poor melodrama such as Maxime Formont's *Le Risque* (1908) the point was adequately made that maternity always posed dangers, though less frequently for the informed middle class than for the workers whom many were trying to keep in ignorance. From the questions of sexual and social inequalities Léon Frapie extended the debate in *La Maternelle* (1905) by pointing out that in addition to the health of the mother the happiness of existing children was endangered by unlimited pregnancies.

> One is continuously beaten over the head with the assertion of "the
> rights of the father of a family," but who will oppose everyone in
> demanding rights for the child? The child not only has the right not to be
> poisoned with alcohol, and not to be poisoned with enslaving beliefs, but
> he bears within him the essential demand *of not having too many
> brothers and sisters.* . . . Here are little girls, aged at thirteen, literally
> used up by the care of brats. This one, Josephine Guépin, who is coming
> to fetch her sister and two brothers, I have never met without a child at
> her hand and another clinging to her skirt; she is finished, her back bent,
> her shoulders bowed. She stops for a moment with her mouth open
> before speaking, the time to heave a sigh, and, her eyes lifeless, tells me
> sincerely, without spite: Mama doesn't mind having children, *I'm the
> one who bears all the burdens.*[41]

As daring as Frapie was in setting the rights of children against those of
parents, his work was not as shocking as the novels in which the issue of
abortion was broached. The actual employment of contraceptives hardly
lent itself to literary depiction, but the drama of a woman faced with the
difficult decision of whether or not to abort naturally attracted a few hardy
novelists. The feminist Jeanne Caruchet in *L'Ensemencée* (1902)
sympathetically presented a woman futilely trying abortifacients,
eventually bearing her child, and ending up bitter and defeated. In André
Vesnière's fascinating account of the sewing trade, *Camille Frison:
Ouvrière de la coutume* (1908), a seduced seamstress ponders the
question of whether to abort or to bear and then abandon her child. She
decides at last to keep it. As much as novelists courageously provided
arguments legitimating the woman's right to abort, they rarely dared to
present the heroine's actually going through with the act. A plot device that
allowed authors to "have it both ways" consisted of presenting the heroine
and a secondary character — usually a servant — both becoming
unexpectedly pregnant but only the latter being made to pay the full price.
In Marcel Tinayre's *L'Ombre de l'amour* (1909), for example, the
pregnant servant girl commits suicide; her mistress, who allows her
pregnancy to go to full term, bears a child which conveniently dies.
Gilberte, the heroine of Ferri-Pisani's *Sterilité* (1906), finds that both she
and her servant have to seek the services of the same abortionist. The
servant has her miscarriage successfully induced, but Gilberte is prevented
by a police raid. The novel does end with another convenient death — that
of Gilberte's husband — which allows her to marry her lover and father of
the baby (a man who, coincidentally, has just been elected deputy on a
proabortion platform) and finally have her child. In the last pages she is
shown "gently, gently, very gently rocking he who had been her greatest

enemy."[42] The contorted nature of the plots of such works naturally limited their artistic success, but their obvious failings as works of literature should not blind one to the daring and determination of their authors. The obvious argument of all these didactic novels was that some form of contraception had to be made available to the masses. What is remarkable about these works is not the often clumsy way in which the issue of abortion was handled, but the very fact that the subject was broached at all. The appearance of such a literature was yet another indication of the extent to which the fertility debate sparked by Robin's activities had become by 1914 a topic of public concern.

Was an obvious "type" attracted to the birth control campaigns of Robin and Humbert? They did seem to be drawn predominantly from the shadowy margins of respectable political and literary life and were often already well prepared by their anarchism or anticlericalism, their anticolonialism or antimilitarism, their feminism or bohemianism, to defend yet another unpopular cause. Some were from modest backgrounds and did not shrink from attacking the status quo, some — as the plethora of noms de plume suggests — saw themselves at war with society and had already gone half undergound; some had not had traditional family lives and felt little reluctance in challenging "normal" sex roles: Gabriel Giroud, Urbain Gohier, and "Libertad" were orphans; Eugène Humbert and Jean Marestan were illegitimate. On the one hand, conservatives, by standing aloof from the birth control campaign, allowed it to be taken over by the libertarians, but on the other, the radicals seized what they took to be a weapon with which to beat the establishment. What was the result of this curious alliance of neo-Malthusians and political radicals? One of its unexpected consequences was that France produced a unique birth control movement that offered a critique of both sexual and political power and called for both the right to abortion and social revolution. In countries such as the United States and Britain the birth control movement was captured by middle-class reformers and philanthropists and turned to the purposes of social control. In France, however, birth control was presented as a weapon in the class and sex struggles.

PART FOUR

The Response

CHAPTER EIGHT

The Working-Class Family and Fertility Control

The fertility debate that raged in the late nineteenth century between neo-Malthusians and sex radicals on the one side and doctors, priests, and moralists on the other was primarily sparked by concern for the reproductive habits of working-class men and women. The purpose of this chapter will be to gauge the influence of the birth control campaign on urban workers. In the following chapters attention will be shifted from class to sex divisions by examining the differences in attitudes of men and women to the problems posed by childbearing.

The first point to be made in any discussion of the effectiveness of Robin's birth control campaign is that observers on both sides appeared to assume that by the 1890s the middle classes could not be forced or cajoled into returning to a tradition abandoned almost a century earlier of raising large families. In *Précis du cours d'économie politique* (1878) Paul Cauwès regretted that although Malthus did not approve of "practiques immorales" his doctrine had led the bourgeoisie to restrict their family size.

> Too abstract to have any effect on the uncultivated minds of the laboring classes, what it [Malthus's doctrine] teaches could be only too easily listened too, but in the wrong way, by the wealthy classes.[1]

Cauwès' concern was that although foresight could not be taught to the poor, an undue concern for security led the rich — whose influence was needed for the health of society — to limit the number of their offspring. In *Mon oncle Benjamin* written in 1881 Charles Tillier presented a character complaining that:

> Women no longer reproduce as they should; these ladies are mothers as infrequently as possible; because of thrift they make themselves sterile. When the wife of the clerk has produced her little clerk, the wife of the notary her little notary, they believe they have paid their dues to the human race and they stop. . . . The fact is that children are very expensive, and this cost is not within the grasp of everyone; only the poor can permit themselves the luxury of a large family.[2]

Emile Faguet in a work aptly entitled . . . et l'horreur des responsabilités
(1911) went much further than Cauwès and Tillier in reprimanding the
bourgeoisie. Faguet asserted that the real family was the large family, the
little tribe, but now fathers of six were considered "des prodigues, des
dissapateurs, des dilapidateurs." Because of their arranged marriages,
bourgeois spouses only grew to love one another through their children;
because they loved their children too much, he said, they had fewer of
them. The nightmare of the middle-class man was, Faguet claimed, to
have more than two children, and indeed, if the first was a son the husband
would want to stop there. The product of such a union would be a spoiled,
egotistical, jealous, passive being, ill-equipped to defend France against the
prolific Italians, Germans, or even the French Jews — the métèques —
who endangered France.[3] But if moralists expressed their anguish at the
decline in natality of the better classes, they had little in the way of specific
suggestions for countering the trend. Clearly, the bourgeoisie could not be
coerced.

Paul Bureau struck the pose of the typically concerned social
commentator when in a report that attributed the fall of working-class
fertility to an aping of middle-class behavior, he went out of his way to
reassure his readers that he did not condemn the latter. "I am not playing
politics and am not attacking anyone, but you will appreciate that this is a
delicate situation."[4] When the same commentators turned to the petite
bourgeoisie and lower classes, it was similarly taken for granted that
because inheritance laws threatened to divide the farm of the peasant with
a large family into tiny portions, the rural propertied population would also,
with the exception of remote Catholic zealots, limit its fertility. As early as
the late eighteenth century it was reported in the Garonne that "one
considers it as a duty to limit one's family."[5] In Normandy in the 1830s M.
Legrand wrote to Antoine Passy, "Thrift is carried to such a degree that
families are careful not to have more than a few children." Fifty years later
Henri Baudrillart wrote of the same province, "Unfortunately, the
voluntary restriction of the number of children has systematic defenders.
There are few who practice it who do not raise it to a point of principle, do
not glorify it as a duty."[6]

By the turn of the century even the most remote regions were
penetrated by Malthusian mores. Actual birth control practices were
sometimes accompanied by the employment of traditional magic
remedies. In Perigord women carried out a "dry mass" to prevent
themselves from conceiving too quickly, in the Nivernais wives beat
themselves with willow bows and in the Vendée drank cups of rue to
obtain the same prophylactic effect.[7] This fear of the large family was made
clear in the proverbs of provincial France. An English traveler reported in

1861, "The cautious French apply the saying, 'Make the soup make the child.'"[8] Jacques Bertillon found that in Nor expressions were, "Desire of a king; a boy and a girl" and "T more than a dozen," that in the Côte d'Or a third child was Désiré, and that in the Orne the parents of large families if they were not, asserted Dr. Rommel, a cause for laughter, were referred to as, "Those people, they are worse than animals."[9]

The real issue posed by the turn-of-the-century fertility debate was, therefore, whether or not the urban working class would follow the pattern of small families set by the middle classes and peasantry. The high fertility norm of the manufacturing class had for much of the century been sustained by the demands for child labor. It was rational for the worker to have a large family when children could be put out to work at an early age. In 1896 Zaborowski, in responding to Paul Robin's defense of birth control, declared:

> It is sufficient to look around us to become assured that, with the exception of rare chance and exceptionally high wages, the workman's family does not reach comfort until after having reared its children. Whatever it may do besides — to rear its children is the surest means, if not the only means, of assuring bread to these old people.[10]

In other words, Zaborowski was stating that in lieu of any form of social security workers had to see their high fertility as a form of old age insurance. The argument made by the birth controllers was that changing social and economic conditions now made the adoption of a strategy of controlled fertility a more reasonable option.

Were the workers who were the targets of Robin's and Humbert's propaganda actually reached? As indicated in previous chapters, the leading socialist and anarchist writers were hostile to the neo-Malthusian campaign and this would no doubt have dissuaded some militants from listening to the birth controllers. That so many bohemians and freethinkers rallied to the cause may also have alienated the more conservative and deferential portions of the working class. But not all arguments in favor of fertility control came from outside the labor movement. The real strength of Robin's campaign lay in rallying to its side many of the leading syndicalists. The left in France was divided in the first decades of the twentieth century between a political movement represented in the Assembly from 1905 on by a unified socialist party led by Jaurès and an industrial movement represented by the Confédération générale du travail (C.G.T.), which repudiated parliamentary activity and advocated a revolutionary syndicalism that would theoretically culminate in a General Strike. Between 1906 and 1910 France was swept not just by waves of strikes aimed at smashing the capitalist state but by the growing interest of the labor movement in formulating its own culture. Maxime Leroy provided a sort of social anthropology of this syndicalist world in *La Coutume ouvrier* (1913). What the syndicalists sought was worker independence, which they saw as being best obtained via the trade union rather than through reliance on traditional forms of political activity. Indeed, the revolutionary syndicalists called for the destruction of the bourgeois state and it was in this context, reported Leroy, that they complemented their antiparliamentarianism and antimilitarism with the defense of birth control. For the most sanguine, the "grève de ventre" was presented as a facet of the General Strike inasmuch as it deprived capitalists of labor; for the more moderate, birth control was presented as a basic means of improving the health and well-being of the working-class family and so a way of preparing workers for the Revolution.[11] That both left- and right-wing politicians attacked restriction of fertility as unpatriotic only served to confirm the suspicions of syndicalists that all deputies were inherently hostile to ordinary workers seeking to control their own destinies.

Support for Robin and Humbert came from the highest level of the syndicalist movement. Leaders of the C.G.T. like Emile Pouget and Victor Griffuelhes showed themselves to be sympathetic; Georges Yvetot actively campaigned at the bourses du travail in favor of small families.[12] Within the trade unions neo-Malthusianism was not without its critics; Alfred Rosmer, for example, attacked the doctrine in *Voix ouvrier*. Defenders appeared, however, even in the columns of *Voix ouvrier* and included Charles Desplanques, a C.G.T. organizer and contributor to *La Voix du peuple;* Louis Grandidier, Dreyfusard and secretary of the Bourse du travail of Saint Denis; V. Franchet, leader of the Syndicats des cuisiniers; and Ernest Verliac who left his post as secretary of the Fédération des métaux to lead the Fédération des ouvriers néo-Malthusien. Arguments in favor of birth control were presented to the Congrès confédéral de Bourges in 1904 by the Fédération des mineurs de Pas-de-Calais and the Bourse du travail of Saint Denis, and repeated at the 1909 Congrès des syndicats de la voiture, the 1905 and 1909 Congrès de la Fédération des cuirs et peaux, the 1909 and 1910 Congrès de la fédération du tonneau, the 1910 Congrès de la fédération de batiment, and the 1911 Congrès de la céramique. On the local level syndicalist support for fertility control was voiced by the Fédération des industries du papier, the Fédération national des ouvriers coiffeurs, the Fédération national de la voiture, the Union des syndicats de la Seine and the Indre, the Jeunesse syndicaliste de Brest and Le Mans, the Syndicat des égoutiers de la Seine, the Union du bronze, the Syndicat des graveurs ciseleurs sur tous métaux, the Syndicat des découpeurs estampeurs de Paris, and the Syndicat des coupeurs et brocheurs en chaussures.[13]

In Paris at the grass-roots level the activists of *Génération consciente* had their propaganda complemented by the more self-consciously proletarian Group ouvrier néo-malthusien (G.O.N.M.), formed in 1910 under the leadership of Ernest Verliac.[14] A sense of this diffusion of neo-Malthusian ideas can be gained by perusing the columns of *Humanité* in which announcements appeared for meetings of sections of *Génération consciente* in Boulogne-Billancourt, in the fourteenth and in the twentieth arrondissements while the G.O.N.M. met in Saint Denis and Puteaux-Nanterre. At the latter local on 6 March 1909 one could hear "Conférence par Cudot de l'union syndicale des ouvriers sur métaux sur le néo-malthusianisme," and on 15 January 1910 in the nineteenth arrondissement " 'Révolution et malthusianisme' par le camarade Philippe et 'Hygiène de la femme' par la citoyenne Scot."[15] In the provinces the authorities noted that the industrial centers of Roubaix, Tourcoing, Le Creusot, Armentières, and Fougères had especially active neo-Malthusian propagandists. In Roubaix they included Jules Blouet, Georges Deveux, and Victor Cornil, who distributed information from a cabaret. In Fougères the local propagandist was an old anarchist by the name of Forthomme, who was aided in 1907 by Léon Marinot while on a speaking tour of the west. Forthomme was the subject of a judicial inquiry in 1911 as were twenty-six reputed abortionists of Tourcoing in 1908. Other provincial propagandists harried by the authorities included Camille Cauvin, prosecuted in Marseilles in 1912, Emile Hamelin, a pacifist jailed in Trelazé, and Jules Le Gall, a syndicalist worker in the Brest arsenal and contributor to the *Prolétaire breton*, arrested in 1907 for a birth control talk. Their efforts were matched by Antoine Antignac, a follower of Sébastien Faure in Bordeaux, Barbe who worked for the Ligue in the Pas de Calais, Croizet who did the same in Lorient, Mme. Jean Dubois in Versailles, Dumenil in Le Havre, a printer named Charles Grasz in the Ain, Mme. Papillon in Lyon, the C.G.T. representative of the "métallurgistes du Boucau" (Basses-Pyrénées) Denis Recolin, Gaston Ville in Rouen, and Dr. Fernand Elosu, anarchist, pacifist, and teetotaler in Bayonne.[16] Prefects reported that workers were being deluged with contraceptive information. The movement's "star" speakers held forth before audiences at bourses du travail, in school yards, in *maisons du peuple*, and even in the town halls of some lax officials. Those who did not attend could read the same message in books, brochures, and articles in the syndicalist press. Neo-Malthusian slogans were also found on gummed stickers, post cards, and wrapping paper used by itinerant peddlers. When workers left their shops in Lyon, Roubaix, and Paris, they had material handed to them;

when they posted their banns of marriage more information came by mail; and if they attended union fêtes at Saint Cloud or Montreaux, they could read on the balloons released at the end of the day the slogans "Maternité consciente" and "grève de ventres."[17]

The syndicalists not only provided a network of agents, journals, and meeting halls by which birth control information could be distributed; they also passed on their advice in a language far more accessible to the worker than that of the dry studies produced by academics of France's demographic situation. For example, in an early account of "le dépopulage" that appeared in Pouget's *Père Peinard* in 1893 the author asserted:

> The assholes who exploit the people constantly shout in our ears or else scrawl in their filthy rags: "The country is being depopulated: the number of births is decreasing!" . . . Listen, this crap is all I hear. But as for us, the exploited and the cheated, do we give a fuck? On the contrary, for God's sake, nothing could be nicer and I even recommend to my pals a general strike in the production of brats.[18]

Those "richards" who bewailed the fall in natality were, claimed the contributor, only shedding crocodile tears. All they wanted was "l'abondance des prolos" because the wives of the bourgeoisie — "putains" and "garces" — only ever had two children themselves . . . "le reste est escamoté." In conclusion the author called on the workers to follow the middle class in having only one or two "mioches" so that one could carry on the Revolution without "derrière soi des piolées des mioches" and leave to one's children a better future than "le dépôt des mendingos pour leur vieux os."

Similar sentiments were carried in poems and songs written for a popular audience. Jehan Rictus in *Le Coeur populaire* warned his readers that revolutionary action in the unions had to be matched by reforms in the home.

> Et c'est parfait les syndicats;
> Mais si tes fess's sont au caca,
> Tu auras des idées merdeuses.[19]

The revolutionary poet J.B. Clément presented the woman's point of view in "Ne me fais plus d'enfants" in which a working-class wife addresses her spouse:

> Ça va venir dans la semaine
> J'ai mal dans les reins et partout.
> Sans espoir tu meurs à la peine
> Et quant à moi, je suis à bout.

Nous sommes déjà six à table
A vivre sur tes quatre francs
Allons, mon vieux, sois raisonnable
Ne me fais plus d'enfants.[20]

An anonymous little song in circulation near Caen in 1915 returned to the theme of bourgeois hypocrisy in the refrain:

Citoyens, disent des gens fort sages
(Deputés, ministres et savants. . .)
Montrez un peu plus de courage,
Au pays donnez des enfants!
Messieurs les heureux de la terre,
Des gosses vous n'en voulez pas
Quand vos bell's dames à manières
S'deform'nt, ell's font vite passer ça.[21]

Here again, a songster succeeded by playing on class hostility in presenting the "population question" in terms immediately intelligible to a working-class audience.

How did the urban working class respond to this barrage of propaganda in favor of birth control? The fall in its fertility could be taken as one sign that the campaign was successful. Such was, not surprisingly, the conclusion of *Génération consciente* and the *Malthusien*. But firsthand accounts of working-class discussions of family strategies indicated that access to contraceptive information was only part of the explanation for falling fertility. The decline in heavy industry, the rise of the service sector with the dramatic entry of women into white-collar work, the continuing reduction of infant mortality, the growth of state interest in the welfare and education of children, and the elimination of children from the work force and the resulting extension of their years of dependence upon parents all contributed to adoption of a small-family strategy.

Children who once were viewed as a valuable economic resource came to be viewed as a burden in overcrowded, working-class tenements. Maurice Beaufreton reported in *Le logement populaire à Paris* (1898): "The worker who does not want to become a tramp has scarcely any other choice than neo-Malthusianism or the slum."[22] The child was not only prevented from working in its early years; the presence of even one child could effectively prevent the mother from contributing to the family wage as the laws restricting women's work came into force. Doctors du Mesnil and Mangenot found in their census of workers' homes in Ivry that 26 percent had no children, 23 had one, 19 percent had two and only 15 percent had three. Why this small size?

Those who have no children told us, "We would really like to have them but we would not be able to feed them." Or else: "If my wife were pregnant, she could no longer work and would therefore be obliged to care for the children." Those who have two or three replied, "The burden that we have assumed is already too heavy, we could not increase it; it would require depriving ourselves of everything."[23]

To the investigators' claim that children were not such a financial charge — that they could be cared for at the crèche from birth to age three, from three to five at the "école maternelle," and finally at the "école primaire" — workers responded:

"Yes, all that is true," they replied, "but it is necessary to feed them at night, give them a bed, provide them with clothes and shoes etc. And then, how is one to have a little happiness with five or six children at one's back?"[24]

Dr. René Martial uncovered in his investigations the same desire of families of modest means to improve their conditions. The law of 2 November 1892 which restricted female and child labor, he found, only forced workers to reappraise the question of family limitation. "But I have heard many times in the working-class world of Paris: 'We don't want any more children if they must lead the same lives as us!'"[25] Martial drew some comfort from the fact that many laborers were ignorant of how they could put their plans into practice; du Mesnil and Mangenot had discovered the same ignorance. After commenting on families with only one or two children, they noted that "other households ingenuously admitted to us that if they had so many children, it was because they did not know how not to have them."[26] Madeleine Vernet believed that there was a great deal of confusion concerning the effectiveness of contraception. A woman worker on being asked why her family was small replied confidently that they took "precautions," but a male laborer retorted, " 'Oh! declara ce camarade, les préservatifs, voyez vous, c'est de la blague!'"[27]

The male worker's remark reminds one that the two sexes did not always regard conception in the same light. Obviously a pregnancy posed more burdens and dangers to the woman than to the man, which explains why many husbands left the question of family planning to their wives, an issue to which we will return in following chapters. Here it might only be noted that such an indifference or stoicism would prevent the rapid diffusion of contraception in working-class areas. A young working-class woman asked in 1904 why she had so many children replied that it was her husband's doing. "He is young and it seems that the tubercular are really carried away by 'it.' Can I refuse him this pleasure which costs me nothing?"[28] The relationship of the fear of tuberculosis to the dislike of employing contraceptives is obscure but apparently was made by the working class throughout Europe. In England at about the same time another woman attributed her pregnancy to the fact that her husband "said it was his rights, and he'd have consumption if we took any precautions. He said that's what always gives men consumption. And now I'm like this!"[29] Some working-class men, moreover, viewed their ability to impregnate as an indication of their masculinity and violently opposed any interference in the matter. Writing to *Régénération* in 1902, a mother painted a painful picture of a slum household in which each sexual encounter was a source of terror.

> My husband saw that I wanted to cheat nature. He flew into an awful rage; I was afraid that he would kill me; I resigned myself to the ordeal and now I am going to live with the continual fear of a fifth child.[30]

Most workers felt compassion for their wives, but given their wretched living conditions which held little hope for improvement, it was hardly surprising that many working couples when asked why they did not control themselves would ask in turn, "Que voulez-vous, nous n'avons que ce plaisir là pour nous."

It was partly in response to such fatalism that Robin and Humbert launched their propaganda campaigns, and from what Martial reported their efforts were meeting with some success:

> They go to the people, make speeches, and indicate the practical ways in which to avoid having children. I, myself, have seen at the door of a factory a street vendor at the lunchtime break selling devices capable of preventing conception. This active propaganda has been going on, to my knowledge, from at least 1899.[31]

Evidence that workers valued such information and resented those who attempted to keep them in ignorance of it can be found in the letters to the editor of the only widely circulated socialist paper which supported the neo-Malthusians — Gustave Hervé's *La Guerre sociale*. More an anticlerical and antimilitarist than a socialist, Hervé initially supported the birth-control movement and ran advertisements for works on contraception in his publication. In 1914, however, with the threat of war emerging, he swung round to the nationalist side and attacked those who preached the restriction of family size. He attempted to disarm syndicalist critics in advance by declaring that he understood that workers were suspicious of the state and church's hypocritically calling for large families; it was a crime to bear children one could not support. Hervé called for a family of three to four children, not in the name of the country or Catholicism but for "la patrie révolutionnaire." France was dying because of the spread of contraception, this "phylloxéra de la race française," an assertion Hervé backed up with references from Leroy-Beaulieu and Boverat indicating that at present levels of natality France would have its population reduced to thirty-two million by 1951. The birth controllers called Hervé "Père Lapin"; Hervé responded by calling them "pères capotes, pères baudruches." He further suggested that their fixation on contraception blinded them to the ultimate catastrophe posed by Germany's might. "The metaphysics of rubber has placed such a blindfold over their eyes that it makes it impossible for them to understand the immediate dangers that this loss of equilibrium between France and the other nations poses to all of us."[32] Judging by the letters Hervé received, few readers were willing to follow his line of argument. His readers accused him of now being a "lapiniste," and he admitted he was scoffed at in syndicalist circles. One correspondent reported just being able to raise two children on eight francs a day and asked how he was supposed to support four. A father of eight lamented the poverty of families deprived of birth control information and reminded Hervé that the real enemies of the people were the populationists like deputy Edme Piot. "Oh, how I would like to have the pleasure of shutting the traps of all the Piots and all the little Piots with shovelfuls of s . . . !"[33]

There seems little doubt that the campaign in favor of birth control played some role in reducing French fertility at the turn of the century, but the precise effect is impossible to determine. Those who went the furthest in attributing the decline to the efforts of Robin, Humbert, and their followers were usually those most intent on outlawing such activities. Paul Bureau testified to the impact that neo-Malthusian speakers had on working-class audiences. When he defended the need for a growing population, he was frequently bitterly attacked by propagandists who impressed workers with demonstrations of the impossibility of raising five or six children on three to five francs a day.[34] The demographer Jacques Bertillon called such lessons "criminal propaganda" that could be ultimately traced back to the "sick brain" of Paul Robin.[35] Boverat accused the neo-Malthusians of depriving France in 1913 of 250,000 souls.[36] The Année sociale internationale tried to provide some statistical support for such a claim by reviewing the decline in births in the provincial cities where the neo-Malthusians had been most active. In Tourcoing the birth rate dropped from 34 per thousand in 1889–1893 to 19 per thousand in 1907–1908, in Roubaix from 32 per thousand in 1889–1893 to 21 per thousand in 1907–1908, in Le Creusot from 30 per thousand in 1893 to 19.7 per thousand in 1904.[37] Of course, all of this was circumstantial evidence and, produced as it was by hostile witnesses, must be used with caution. It does seem safe to say that the neo-Malthusians made information available to some workers and women previously left in ignorance, but whether or not such new knowledge was put into practice depended on both social context and individual circumstances. That workers were far more interested in the practical consequences of family limitation than with the ideology which accompanied it was made clear by a working woman when asked by Senator Béranger whether she was influenced by the neo-Malthusian propaganda. She responded,

> "We are our own mistresses!" And then I asked her: "Have you read this little paper?" She said to me: "I read it, I understand nothing in it. In the books that are sold us it is impossible to understand anything, but it is for the illustrations and for the addresses that are at the back that one buys them."[38]

CHAPTER NINE

Abortion as Birth Control

What role did women play in France's nineteenth-century birth control debate? In this chapter we will deal with actual measures taken by wives and mothers to control their fertility. This discussion will thus provide a backdrop for the following chapter's examination of the feminist response to the issue. Extended discussion of women's thoughts and actions are, of course, warranted because women were obviously more directly affected than men by the availability or lack of contraceptive information. A series of unwanted pregnancies could result in ill health and even death. But reliance upon contraception was not the only way to limit family size; abortion, which has been largely ignored by demographers, also played an important role. Quantifiers are no doubt put off by the difficulty, if not the impossibility, of accurately establishing the incidence of acts that were illegal and therefore hidden from public scrutiny. It would appear, however, that the reluctance of historians and demographers to discuss even the possible importance of abortion is also due to an unwillingness to accept the notion that women could play an active part in determining family size. Demographic theory has in general held that coitus interruptus was the main, initial means of contraception. In other words it has been assumed that the restriction of family size was primarily the consequence of male decisions and actions. Wrigley, for example, states:

> It may be of some importance that coitus interruptus is essentially a male
> act since in animal populations in general the social activities which serve
> to maintain populations near an optimum are normally a male preserve.[1]

As we have seen, there can be little doubt that, except for abstinence, coitus interruptus was the earliest and simplest form of contraception. What seems to be forgotten is that it was also unreliable. If a couple intent on limiting the size of their family were to rely solely on the withdrawal method, there was a good chance that eventually a "mistake" would be made. What then? I would argue that the couple now would have to contemplate the option of abortion as a backup method of fertility control. In other words, once the male method had failed the female method would be employed.[2]

If one examines nineteenth-century discussions of France's declining birth rate, one discovers that commentators attributed a key role to abortion. Whereas in the first half of the century the practice was viewed primarily as an exceptional act, the last resort of the unwed mother, in the latter half it was increasingly acknowledged as a married woman's backup method of birth control. Given the nature of the documentation available, it is difficult to determine if women were in fact having recourse to abortion more frequently than in the past, but the increased reportage of such measures does cast a fresh light on the medical profession's attitudes toward the general problem of fertility control. Doctors assumed that as efforts to limit family size with the use of unreliable contraceptives expanded, so too would recourse to abortion. They acknowledged that surgeons were themselves responsible for making abortion a "thinkable" option because on a practical level they had showed it could be accomplished within relative margins of safety. They accepted the notion that the abortion issue posed the crucial question of whether the woman's control of her own body was an individual right or a selfish, antisocial act.

The following discussion will attempt to place the abortion issue in its nineteenth-century context. Two words of warning. First, regarding sources, I have had to rely to a large extent on medical accounts of women's sexual behavior. Doctors were obviously the best-placed male observers to comment on abortion, but they were in the main violently opposed to the practice being carried out by nonmedical personnel. Their reports are thus necessarily biased and the way in which this might affect the chapter's argument will have to be considered. Second, this chapter has to be, because of the questionable nature of the quantifiable materials, restricted almost solely to *attitudes* toward abortion. Little will be said concerning the actual incidence of the practice. Nevertheless, central to the argument is the assumption that ideas both reflect and influence actions. The belief that control of family size was possible, that inducement of miscarriage could be safely performed, that a woman had the right to choose whether or not to bear a child — all of these issues surfaced in the latter half of the nineteenth century. That such ideas should be articulated at a particular time provides perhaps only a distorted picture of reality, but given the nature of the problem, it is likely the only picture we shall be able to obtain.

Recourse to abortion did not begin with the nineteenth century. References to the practice can be found as far back in French history as one cares to look. In 1566 Henri Estienne referred to midwives being brought to private homes to provide abortions.[3] The famous seventeenth-century royal *sage-femme* Louise Bourgeoise warned her daughter in *Instruction à ma fille* that if she were to allow women to use her home when lying-in she would be suspected of acting as an abortionist.[4] In the eighteenth century the practice was noted by Montesquieu, Rousseau, and de Sade.[5] The pioneer demographer Moheau exclaimed in 1773: "What risks children run! Before they are born their mothers often form against them homicidal plans; pity those whose mothers are instructed in the art of early murders."[6] For the purpose of this chapter what is most interesting in the reports of abortion is the change that takes place in the nineteenth-century representation of the type of woman who would seek to induce her own miscarriage. In the first half of the century the assumption was frequently made that she would be a widow or unmarried woman attempting to avoid bearing an illegitimate child; in the second half it was increasingly acknowledged that married women were adopting the practice as a form of fertility control.[7] The evidence does not suggest that there was in fact a clear break in practices; the shift in attention reflected rather an evolution in the general attitude toward restriction of family size.

In the early nineteenth century the abortion question surfaced as part of the general debate over the purposes of the foundling homes. The number of *enfants abandonnés* increased from 84,000 in 1815 to 127,000 in 1833. Much of this increase was attributed by critics to the lax admission policy — in particular the *tours*, the turntables at doors of the foundling homes, which allowed a mother to deposit a child unobserved.[8] The baron de Gerando in *Le visiteur du pauvre*, a text awarded in 1820 the prize of the Lyon Academy as the best work on charity, saw the homes as necessary only to the extent that they prevented the infanticide of illegitimate children. They were to be simply repositories for the "fruit de la séduction ou de la débauche."[9] He was concerned by the fact that the tours also permitted the abandonment of large numbers of legitimate children. The homes were thus open to attack as providing an easy solution for parents too lazy and immoral to raise their own children.

With the coming of the July Monarchy those economists imbued with English, laissez-faire, Malthusian ideas led an all-out assault on the homes. Duchatel, Blanqui, and others argued that if the tours were not closed a bounty would be held out to the promiscuous and the improvident.[10] A popular piece of propaganda put out by these economists was that a poor mother would leave her child at the home at night and turn up the next morning to offer her services as a paid nurse for her own offspring — a stratagem similar to that carried out by Moses' mother but which nevertheless horrified nineteenth-century economists.

The defenders of the tours argued that to restrict the assistance offered to impoverished mothers would not improve morality. If children could not be left, women would be forced to abortion or infanticide. Such acts were not defended but presented as inevitable consequences of the state's heartlessness. Alphonse Esquiros pointed out the contemptuous opinion of women held by the economists.

> One of the constraints that nature has put on the libertinage of women, say the adversaries of the tour, is the fear of having children: to teach them to brave such a peril is to destroy the dike that holds back most of them from depraved penchants.[11]

Such beliefs, declared Esquiros, were both unworthy and shortsighted. The real question was whether or not infant life was or was not to be protected. The defenders of the tours held that when they were closed the infanticide rate went up. The socialist François Vidal stated in 1846:

> The tours have been closed and the poor mother, the working-class girl has been left no other option than abortion or infanticide. In our sad society many mothers have bewailed their fecundity, and more than one, in thinking of the future which awaits her newborn, has broken its head on the cobbles, or strangled it with maternal hands in order *to deliver it from life*, to spare it misery.[12]

Figures showing that the infanticide rate rose where the tours were closed were advanced by de Girardin, himself illegitimate, in 1846, Viallet in 1847, Tardieu in 1868, and Brochard in 1876.[13] Chatagnier, a judge at Bourg, concurred and added that in those areas where the infanticide rate did not go up it was because recourse was made to abortion.[14] Dr. H.E. Dutouquet stated in 1866 that upon the closing of the tours "the private lying-in homes are too often abortion shops."[15] According to Brochard, "the number of infanticides is immense, the number of abortions incalculable."[16] M. de Bethman *administrateur des enfants trouvés* at Bordeaux, was quoted as saying that:

> infanticides have increased, because of the difficulties experienced by unwed mothers seeking the admission of their children [to the foundling homes]; abortions are of an unheard-of frequency, almost a habit; to the extent that a large number of midwives, lower level practitioners, make no scruple in lending their assistance to poor seduced girls and thus save them from dishonor.[17]

To cite Brochard once more:

> Abortion, unfortunately, is not considered a crime it is a *social practice*. Who has not seen married women regretting a pregnancy, for them undesired, and bitterly complaining of it? From the regret to the abortion is only a step, and this step is often taken by married women. How can it

not be taken by unfortunate young girls who see on one side shame, on the other safety?[18]

The references made to abortion in the literature defending the tours is of great interest, but since they form part of a polemic they must be treated with some caution.[19] It is not unlikely, for example, that the rates of infanticide and abortion would be exaggerated by men who sought to prove that such acts were a consequence of the harsh policies implemented by their opponents. Yet the assumptions made by these observers are striking. It was assumed that knowledge of abortive practices was widespread and that even married women had recourse to them. It was assumed that the public at large would sympathize perhaps not with a married woman freeing herself from a legitimate pregnancy, but with a seduced girl, prevented by the law that forbade the *récherche de paternité* from having the support of the father of the child and faced with the alternatives of abortion or social ostracization. The fact that most women arrested for abortion were single seemed to confirm the argument that the practice was only a last resort of the unmarried.

Up to the middle decades of the nineteenth century the popular image of the type of woman seeking an abortion was that of the seduced girl; from the 1880s on it was that of the married woman seeking to control the size of her family. This shift appears to have been based on the growing assumption that the desire to limit family size was so great but the effectiveness of contraceptives still so questionable that the married increasingly found recourse to abortion necessary as a second line of defense against undesired pregnancies. The practice was increasingly referred to in the latter half of the nineteenth century no longer as the last resort of the unwed, seduced girl but as a family planning measure employed by the married woman. As a result the nature of the idea and practice of abortion was transformed. Whereas in the case of the single girl, the pregnancy she would seek to terminate would be her first, for the married woman it would be the third or fourth that threatened the family with one child too many. In the first case it was an exceptional act; in the second, part of a couple's plans to limit the family. Abortion had become but one of several methods of birth control. The very fact that a couple had used other methods would prepare them psychologically, should they fail, to fall back on abortion. As the use of contraceptive measures in general increased in the course of the century, so too would the necessity — if the couple was adamant in maintaining the family at a particular size — of contemplating recourse to abortion. Therefore, even though most proponents of birth control in France — as in Britain and America — condemned abortion and indeed argued that it would be eliminated only if contraceptive techniques were more widely known, it was more likely that in the short run the use of both methods of fertility control would rise together.[20]

The employment of contraceptive techniques made the practice of abortion within marriage "thinkable" in two ways. First, if fertility had been controlled for some time, a couple would be psychologically prepared to view family limitation as normal. It was now plausible that an unexpected pregnancy might be greeted as something "abnormal" and thus legitimate to meet with unusual means. The economist Paul Leroy-Beaulieu stated that one act led naturally to the other:

> The logical neo-Malthusians, who draw all the consequences of their doctrine, admit, in the case in which contraceptive practices and artifices of a union of the sexes, due to bad luck, fail, the right of abortion and there are those among them who demand what they call the freedom of abortion.[21]

Second, the fact that the lower classes knew that the upper classes had at their disposal expensive but effective means of contraception provided the poor with a justification for employing means which they might not have chosen but to which they were driven by poverty. In 1913 Paul Bureau noted:

> In fact the people know that Malthusian practices are commonly adopted in certain bourgeois milieux, in the richest milieu, the most comfortable, even in the governmental milieux.[22]

This was confirmed by a working-class woman who wrote the economist Charles Gide in 1909:

> The large majority [of working-class women] are ignorant of the means used, it seems, for a long time by the well-to-do. . . . What they unfortunately too often do is to try to remove the beginnings of a pregnancy. They thus destroy their health.[23]

Recourse to abortion was also made thinkable for the reason that both medical and nonmedical practitioners were claiming by midcentury that it could be carried out in relative safety. Up to this point we have used the term abortion to refer to the act that at the time was labeled a "criminal abortion" to separate it from a "therapeutic abortion." By the middle decades of the nineteenth century French physicians were carrying out the latter operation in those cases where delivery at term posed serious dangers to a mother's health. It might be noted that the justification for such practices took longer to establish in the French medical community than in its British or German counterparts. A line of doctors from

Mauriceau to Fodéré to Cazeaux had to battle with the idea that one should have faith in the resources of nature.[24] On the contrary, these liberal physicians contended that if a mother was endangered by hemorrhaging or convulsions a miscarriage should be induced; if the question was raised as to who should live, the answer was obviously the mother. The Académie de Médecine was appealed to in 1827 by Costa and in 1852 by Cazeaux to formally justify such actions. In each case it refrained.[25] On condition consultations were first made with colleagues it left the decision of whether or not to induce miscarriage to the discretion of the individual doctor.

Some surgeons saw the Caesarean operation as an alternative. Its chief proponent J.L. Baudelocque argued that the Caesarean — "the grandest and most dangerous operation in surgery," inasmuch as not just one but two lives were endangered — offered the doctor a means of saving both mother and child. But to follow this line of argument required closing one's eyes to the staggering death toll the operation entailed.[26] Others simply fell back on the church's injunction — reinforced in the nineteenth century by Dunot de Saint-Maclou, P.J.C. Debreyne, and Cardinal Gousset — that it was a greater sin to kill an innocent child than a sinful adult. Hence it could be argued that it was better that both mother and child die than that the mother, by an induced miscarriage, be saved.[27]

Most doctors were by 1850 apparently sympathetic to the arguments based on a mother's right of self-defense that were advanced by defenders of therapeutic abortion. Once surgeons were convinced that a mother's life was endangered they would induce miscarriage and indeed publicly claimed that it could be done without great difficulty. As far as the argument of this chapter is concerned, the important point is that although doctors continued to be opposed to any other sort of abortion, the success they achieved in therapeutic abortions could only make the practice, even when carried out for different motives, appear possible and therefore thinkable. Dr. Alexandre Gueniot, accoucheur en chef de la Maternité, specifically attributed the increase in the numbers of such acts to what he referred to as the emergence of "la médecine utilitaire."[28]

By mid-century there were in addition numerous professional abortionists who would carry out operations that were not medically justified. The abortionists came from the ranks of doctors, midwives, matrons, pharmacists, herbalists, veterinarians, bonesetters, masseurs and quacks. Dr. Ambroise Tardieu, the chief investigator of nineteenth-century abortion, declared that by the 1860s abortion had become an "industry."[29] At the end of the century Bertillon could report that fifty abortionists were advertising in the Paris papers. Typical announcements read:

"Troubles mensuels. Si inquiet écrivez rue . . . , no . . . "
"Sages femmes . . . Stéril(ité) Discr(étion) Meth(ode) infaillible"
"Retard, moyen infaillible"[30]

Some abortionists employed "de véritables courtiers" who received a commission for each client sent on; others used the "marchands à la toilette" to advertise their service.[31] The Parisian professionals were, according to Gustave Drouineau, clustered near the train stations and the "grands magasins" to provide for women coming up from the country.[32]

The group that was singled out by the investigators as providing the greatest number of abortionists was the midwife profession. It was a commonplace of the 1890s that the *sages-femmes* made more from abortions than from births. Verrier referred to one who carried out a hundred abortions a year at one hundred francs an operation.[33] Madeleine Pelletier stated the fee could range from ten francs to two hundred francs.[34] These were prices the impoverished midwife could turn down only with difficulty. If she could not provide the service herself, she would send the patient on to someone who could. Indeed, Barthélemy attributed much of the "problem" simply to the oversupply of midwives. Already policed by the law of 19 Ventôse, year XI, midwives were further restricted by the statute of 30 March 1892, to assisting only at those births free of all medical complications. In Paris there were sixty thousand births a year but at least half took place in publicly assisted establishments. Thus thirty thousand births remained to be dealt with by one thousand midwives. In one-fourth of the cases, they would be facing the additional competition of approximately four thousand doctors. The upshot was that these midwives could not possibly survive on their earnings and so would have to turn to assisting those women seeking abortion.[35] It was from the ranks of the midwives that came some of the most famous *faiseuses d'anges* (literally "angel makers," the popular late nineteenth-century French expression for abortionists). They included semilegendary figures known by such sobriquets as "Madame Tiremonde," "La Mort Aux Gosses," "La Cacheuse," "Le Plieuse de Mort." The very fact that they enjoyed such notoriety is one indication of the public acknowledgment of their role.[36]

Doctors were eager to denounce the midwife abortionist if only because midwifery itself provided the medical profession with a competitor it was seeking to destroy. There is no doubt, however, that many doctors also turned to abortion.[37] Along with the female faiseuse d'anges one finds references to "L'homme à l'aiguille," and "Le dégringoleur." In the case of doctors the argument was again made that the fees offered were too tempting to spurn. Henri Bérenger in *Les prolétaires intellectuels en France* (1901) stated that the oversupply of physicians in Paris reduced many to the "exercice louche" of abortion. Some doctors were to make a great deal of money in this trade. In 1912 two abortionists were reported to have brought in over 50,000 francs a year.[38]

A good deal of public attention was focused on the professional abortionists, but Tardieu suggested that a woman would likely avail herself of such services only as a last resort. She would first seek to induce her own miscarriage by drinking an infusion of one of the traditional abortifacients such as rue, savine, or ergot of rye. If that failed, she would try bleedings, hot baths, violent exercises, and whatever friends might recommend. Finally, if she were not yet between the third and fifth month when the quickening of the foetus provided a "frein moral" and caused the abandonment of further attempts, she would turn to the abortionists.[39]

> At the first sign [of pregnancy] one runs to the soothsayers, the midwives, the doctors. One take powders, brews of all sort and every kind. One delivers oneself to heavy labors, to criminal maneuvers. Sometimes one even has recourse to the FAISEUSES D'ANGES![40]

Abortion, which had always been an emergency measure, was acknowledged in the latter half of the nineteenth century as a backup measure of birth control. A host of commentators reported an upsurge in its frequency and in particular to abortions induced by married working-class women. In 1855 Dr. Chatagnier wrote that there were households in which abortion was viewed as only an "innocent protection."[41] Mme. La Chapelle declared in 1891 that most women seeking abortion were now married.[42] Dr. Boismoreau reported in 1911 that in the Vendée even the peasant women were seeking to control their fertility by taking each morning "une bonne infusion de rue."[43]

Most contemporary observers believed that there was an obvious relationship between urbanization and industrialization on the one hand, and the rise of abortions on the other. In the cities more women were working outside the home. If a pregnancy threatened to deprive the family of the woman's income, the inducement of miscarriage offered a way out. Working in a factory or workshop, a woman would have the advice of her fellow workers on what methods to follow. C. Granier, Inspecteur Général des Services Administratifs du Ministre de l'Intérieur, noted that abortion required the complicity of others while infanticide was usually the act of the isolated individual; the first was an urban crime, the second rural.[44]

Working-class women did not rely simply on professional abortionists; they helped each other. According to Dr. Chatagnier,

> little girls know the name of the garden plants of their village which provide the poisonous substance. But it is especially in the city that this

scourge carries out its greatest ravages; there, and in certain gatherings, the ending of pregnancies by abortifacients is noted almost daily; friends do not even hide it from each other; it is a thing understood, excused, accepted — "In such a case, what do you take, Eugénie?" "I take this, it is quicker; and you Marie?" "I take that, it is safer." — Here, one knows the wretches who sell drugs, there the midwife who provides other remedies, elsewhere the bonesetter who operates with instruments, elsewhere again the gossips who store up these diverse expedients.[45]

Writing in 1911 Hubert Legrand stated that abortions were:

almost always the work of a neighbor or of a husband. It is currently an operation which is practiced by the working classes without the slightest fear; when the operation has begun the woman is willing to have herself admitted to the hospital and she admits quite openly what has occurred. There are also the very many cases in which women abort themselves. Nothing is easier, moreover, and they know very well how to find out from each other.[46]

The rising abortion rate was not attributed simply to industrial change; it was also taken as a symptom of an emerging feminism. Granier declared in 1906 that feminist theories were leading to a greater sympathy being felt by the public for mothers who aborted.[47] Such was the extent of feminine solidarity that Marcel Bouteiller wrote that around 1900 the women of the village of Louerre in the Maine and Loire put up a lively resistance to the municipal government's plan to chop down "le gros chillou" or old oak tree in the village square because they relied on a "tisane de gui de chêne" as a traditional abortifacient.[48] Drouineau, reporter of the "Commission de la dépopulation," stated in 1908 that a few years earlier women would not have admitted to an abortion but now because of a changing "mentalité féminine," they freely divulged such secrets.[49]

An aspect of this new "mentality" commented on by many observers was an apparent increase in mutual support of woman to woman, midwife to patient, mother to daughter. Madeleine Pelletier described the solidarity of working-class women in the face of unthinking husbands:

The women, besides, do not make a mystery of these [abortive] practices. On the landings of the working-class tenements, at the bakers, the butchers, the grocers, the housewives advise neighbors whose husbands, as brutal as they are shortsighted, inflict on them unwanted pregnancies.[50]

A similar sense of sisterhood was noted in the middle classes by G.M. Savarit, who stated that the bourgeoisie had become so accustomed to small families that "mothers-in-law glower at the son-in-law when they announce the arrival of a second or third child: these sons-in-law are criminals!"[51] Dr. Burlureux confessed in 1909: "More and more we are struck by the astonishing cynicism with which women — many women, and of every class — talk of such practices as the most natural and permissible of acts."[52] He further said that many women openly asked their doctors for help and were shocked when refused. If they induced their own miscarriage and encountered complications, they felt no shame in returning to their physician for aid; they knew his vow of professional secrecy permitted them to tell all.

> One has to hear how freely they relate their adventure, without the shadow of shame or remorse, because they say, "the woman must have the freedom of her body," and, after all, she "hurts no one in freeing herself" since the child which was going to be born was not yet born.[53]

The medical students of Dr. P.A. Lop were warned that every doctor and midwife had to face the prospect of dealing with numerous women who were convinced of the legitimacy of such acts and who frequently had the support of their husbands.[54]

A third reason advanced by contemporaries to explain the upsurge of abortion was the belief that it was no longer dangerous. In 1913 Barthélemy declared:

> The preservation of the race has been protected for a long time by the fear of danger. This sentiment has disappeared! Today one can procure an abortion just as one has a tooth extracted. It is nothing, it is done so quickly, with so few risks! This is whispered in the *ateliers*. This is known in all classes of society . . . and the evil spreads.[55]

A. Lacassagne stated that because of the popularization of antiseptic theories abortions met with fewer complications and as a consequence infanticides, in comparison, had by the turn of the century sunk into insignificance.[56] The increased reports of the use of "sondes," speculums, douches, and what were referred to as "canules anglaises" does seem to indicate that women were turning to their own use the hygiene lessons of Pasteur. A self-induced miscarriage was still obviously dangerous. If mechanical means were employed there were the problems of peritonitis and hemorrhaging, but it is difficult to determine the risks involved. The medical profession made no effort to enlighten the public in this area. Indeed, many were convinced that doctors in their zeal to prevent the practice had wildly exaggerated its dangers.[57]

What was not frequently mentioned were the nonmedical dangers of seeking the help of another party in procuring an abortion. Since it was a crime, the woman ran the risk of being blackmailed, especially if she relied on a quack. Moreover, many of the drugs that were sold as abortifacients were quite useless. Here again the purchaser was in no position to prosecute the seller. Finally, more than one doctor was to pride himself on having tricked a woman into carrying her pregnancy to full term. Dr. J.M.P. Munaret, for example, stated that it was his practice to give to those patients who sought abortion simple candy pills while assuring them that all would be well.

> The foetus has the time to grow and strengthen itself while my pills are being used, which makes all the more difficult, dangerous, new attempts at abortion. To save a child from death, and a mother from crime, what could be a more wonderful result?[58]

How many abortions were occurring in the latter half of the nineteenth century? Police figures are of little use because as contemporaries noted, the number of convictions for the act bore no relation to the actual level of the practice.[59] According to Robert Michels, "abortion is so widely practiced today [1914] by married people of all social classes, and is justified by so many excuses, that, as far as may be, the legal authorities shut their eyes to the commission of the offense."[60] An arrest only took place when something went seriously wrong, so if the figures tell us anything it is the incidence of *unsuccessful* abortions. As for the successful, Dr. Brochard stated:

> Abortion and infanticides have never been as numerous as they are today [1876]. The criminal statistics that are ceaselessly invoked to prove the contrary signify absolutely nothing. Abortion and infanticide are the two crimes the easiest to commit and the easiest to hide. Most of the time they are not and cannot be prosecuted.[61]

Tardieu pointed out that the statistics not only gave a false picture of the numbers of women involved, but they also presented a misleading portrayal of the type of woman involved. For example, the number of single women was probably exaggerated for the simple reason that they were more likely to be arrested. A married woman who miscarried raised few suspicions; with a single woman there was the chance of the doctor, neighbors, or even the police investigating. Moreover, in a time of trouble the single woman had fewer resources at her disposal, she had fewer people to whom she could turn, and the likelihood of her arrest was therefore all the greater.[62]

To gauge the extent of recourse to abortion it is necessary to fall back on more reliable accounts than those figures collected by the police. From the former evidence we can sketch out a rough idea of the incidence. Thus in 1890 one abortionist admitted in court to servicing two thousand women; in 1891 another confessed to ten thousand.[63] The tactic of starting an abortion by oneself and then going along to hospital to have it completed appears to have increasingly been adopted at the turn of the century. According to Dr. Henri Roulland of the Hôpital Saint-Antoine:

> Many times I have interrogated women who come to ask us to finish an abortion which has begun or to cure the uterine infection caused by criminal acts. As soon as they are sure that we are bound by professional discretion they are all quite open; some even are proud of their action and declare themselves ready to do it again, not wanting, or not wanting any more, children.[64]

As a result, in 1902 Delbet stated that 7 percent of all women hospital patients were recovering from self-induced abortions; Dr. Doléris quoted the figure 17.7 percent and by 1913 Balthazard raised it to 30 percent. In 1884 Charles Pajot maintained that there were as many abortions in the country as live births. In 1906 Dr. Lacassagne claimed that in Lyon there were 10,000 abortions to 9,000 births. In Paris Robert Monin estimated that 100,000 miscarriages were induced each year. For the nation as a whole, the figure was put at 150,000 by Balthazard, 185,000 by Prevost, and 500,000 by S. du Moriez. Government reports after the war referred to 300,000 to 500,000 miscarriages a year.[65]

Such figures are staggering; did doctors have reasons for exaggerating the problem? Several come to mind. First, doctors who were opposed to *all* forms of fertility control found it politic to attribute the entire short fall in French fertility solely to abortion. Second, doctors hostile to midwives and popular practitioners used these figures as evidence of the need to curtail sharply unsupervised medical practice. Finally, doctors angered by an emerging feminism responded by blaming France's "race-suicide" — not on a decision made by husband and wife — but on the selfish act of the independent woman. Interestingly enough, proabortionists cited the same high figures but for quite different reasons.[66] Their argument was that since abortion was so widespread it had to be legalized and made medically safe. One can only assume that the actual number of abortions carried out lies somewhere between the few dozens noted by the police and the hundreds of thousands claimed by physicians. Even if the figure is placed at 100,000 — an extremely low estimation in the eyes of many commentators in the 1890s — one is still faced with a major social issue.

Given the extent of abortion in France, it was not surprising that a defense of the practice should have been produced here earlier than in either England or Germany. The first fully articulated argument in favor seems to have been E. Adolph Spiral's *Essai d'une étude sur l'avortement* published in 1882.[67] Spiral maintained first that the law was counterproductive. If an unmarried girl were forced to bear a child, her chance of living a normal life would be doomed and her likely fate would be one of poverty, crime, or prostitution. The desperate who could not abort would turn to infanticide. Second, the law was inequitable and class biased. Spiral stated that the working class knew that the bourgeoisie had its own methods of controlling fertility — *les fraudes conjugales* — which were not punished by law. The law was simply aimed at the methods of the poor. Third, many women were forced to abortion by the state itself; in particular by the policies that had closed the tours and forbidden the "recherche de paternité." Therefore, it was necessary to conclude that abortion was in some cases morally justifiable.

> We do not hesitate to say yes, if she acts out of fear of not being able to feed by her own efforts, either herself or her children; we believe that in this way she saves not only herself from dishonor but moreover she renders a great service to society.[68]

Spiral did not believe such a right would be abused. Rather, he was convinced it would lead to transforming an immoral and degraded society into a healthy and law-abiding population.

It was natural that the seduced young woman was Spiral's first concern. Her right to abortion could be accepted by many who had refused that right to the married woman. Auguste Forel of Zürich, for example, cautiously accepted the argument that social as well as health reasons had to be taken into consideration, but he thought that in the final account only rape or the seduction of a minor warranted abortion.[69] It was hoped by many that if the law on the recherche de paternité was changed women could either marry or at least obtain maintenance and thus not be forced to extremes. In the words of Dr. Léon Dumas it was necessary to abrogate either article 317 (the law on abortion) or article 340 (the law forbidding the recherche de paternité).[70]

Others pushed the argument further. Dr. A. Wylm stated in 1907 that the law was too rigid. It made no allowance for whether the girl was raped or not, whether the foetus was viable or not, whether the child would be healthy or not.[71] Some doctors also expressed their concern at the toll in mothers' health being levied by illegal abortions. Abortion was dangerous, stated Naquet and others, because it was secret and uncontrolled. To legalize it would purge it of some of its worst evils, including the fatal operations and criminal prosecution suffered by the poor and unlucky.[72]

The most dramatic arguments in favor of abortion were those that reflected the current of feminist thought of the late nineteenth century. Banks has argued that in Britain feminism and family planning were not supportive ideologies. In France, though it is true that many of the leading feminists avoided becoming involved in the birth control debate, the question of a woman's right to abortion was recognized by several as a crucial issue. As early as 1891 the anarchist Séverine (Caroline Rémy) leaped to the defense of women who had recourse to abortion:

> As long as there will be in the world bastards and hungry children, the flag of Malthus, the flag spattered with the blood of infanticides, will float over this army of rebel amazons who, forced by your laws to keep their breasts dry, have the right to keep their loins infertile.[73]

Jacques Lux noted in 1908 that the flaunting of the abortion law seemed to be accompanied by a growing restlessness of women that he attributed to the feminist ideas percolating through society in the works of writers such as Léon Blum and Ellen Key.[74] In 1904 Dr. Edouard Toulouse defended abortion and stated that women were insisting on freeing themselves from the burdens of motherhood.

> This duty of sacrificing their physical personality to the public interest has in no way been accepted by them and it is in fact a real tax in blood to which women submit without having, as does the man forced to be a soldier, the guaranteed assistance of the state.[75]

Toulouse went on to declare:

> It appears to me to be just that the woman have the right to obtain an abortion when the pregnancy bothers her, frightens her, causes her serious social damage. She must be sole judge in this matter, all the more so inasmuch as she often has been, by imprudence, and not voluntarily and after reflection, placed in this situation.[76]

Dr. Courtault concurred. He stated that if the state could not force a man to support a child then it had no right to force the woman to bear it. The woman had as much right to control her own body as a man. An abortion carried out by a trained practitioner before the fourth month posed no problems and Courtault accordingly called for its legalization.[77]

A full feminist defense of abortion was produced just before the First World War by Dr. Madeleine Pelletier, editor of *La Suffragiste*. Pelletier stated that woman had for ages been used by man for his pleasure. Woman had her own sexual desires and in the future they could be fully expressed in a sort of free love. At the moment she was constrained by lack of economic independence and the burden of childbearing. It was the child who plunged the woman back into subjection. If economic equality had existed between the sexes a pregnancy would not have been a calamity, but even so Pelletier still considered it a woman's right to choose whether to bear the child.

Pelletier saw abortion as a particularly important issue for working-class women. They could not afford the contraceptives of the upper classes, they were not as methodical. They often had to deal with indifferent or brutal husbands. They often simply assumed the responsibility of fertility control. For all these reasons abortion was an important backup method of birth control that had to be legalized.[78]

As far as the bourgeoisie were concerned, Pelletier presented a different picture — not that of the mother with the knowledge and means to protect herself but that of the daughter seeking recourse to abortion.

> Abortion is no longer, as previously, the exception; it is, one can say, the rule, and in all classes of society. Today the young bourgeois girl who makes a *mistake* and becomes pregnant no longer thinks of suicide; she thinks of obtaining an abortion.[79]

"The right thing to do" for the respectable young man involved was to offer to marry her or to help her obtain an abortion. The ultimate decision was the girl's.

The final step in the defense of abortion was taken when writers such as Eugène Brieux, Ferri-Pisani, and Daniel Riche permitted the abortionist herself to express her feelings. In Daniel Riche's *Stérile* (1898) a Madame Martin asks,

> Why am I a wretch? . . . You belong to a class which does not know all the sufferings that result from a large family. You should see, near at hand, the difficulties, the anxiety, and the complications which arise in a crowded room at the arrival of a new existence; you should see the women, their youth destroyed, their strength exhausted, and their lives spoilt by overfatigue, to understand that in the slums many children are a misfortune. You wish to suppress this misery? But you should then teach women not to have children when they are unwilling to have them. If you leave women in ignorance, they will continue to have need of my assistance. As in the case of all that lives, every function has its utility: but when women shall know how to avoid maternity, without any operation, which is always dangerous, they will no longer come to seek our assistance.[80]

Abortion found a number of articulate defenders in the first years of the twentieth century because it was already well established as a means of birth control. What conclusions can we draw from this reappraisal of the practice? First, it has been shown that no discussion of birth control is complete unless the option of abortion is included. It has been argued that a rise in contraceptive practices — if they are not fully effective — will be accompanied by an increase in abortion. In the case of bourgeois women abortion was first a normal backup method but became increasingly unnecessary. For working-class women who, though interested in controlling fertility, were for some time cut off from completely reliable methods, it would be especially important. Indeed, in the absence of safe contraceptives abortion might have been the working woman's only form of protection. Thus the nineteenth-century French experience was to anticipate that of twentieth-century nations passing through the "demographic transition." Second, it has been suggested that the working class was not, as has been traditionally asserted, solely dependent on its social superiors in learning about means of fertility limitation. The general tendency of birth control studies has been to present family planning as an innovation, the knowledge of which trickled down the social hierarchy from the upper to the lower classes. What these studies have overlooked is that for the nineteenth-century working class the questions of fertility, infant and child mortality, and the economic utility of children would all have a bearing on whether or not methods of control were considered. That working-class families remained larger than those of the middle class did not mean that the worker was "ignorant" of the means of family restriction. The higher fertility norm of workers in general was rational given a situation in which children raised frugally and put to work early could be valuable assets. When this ceased to be the case and when pregnancies seriously impeded the woman's ability to work, the decision to restrict family size would be considered. If there were no education to provide or fortune to pass on, the decision would be primarily the woman's concern, especially if she controlled the family budget. And to control fertility she did not wait passively for new information but took advantage of whatever means were already at her disposal, including inducement of miscarriage.

How do these findings relate to the current controversy on the effect of women's employment on fertility? They demonstrate that the working class did not depend, as Edward Shorter contends, on hearing from the middle class the "good news" that family limitation was possible. They also lead one to suggest that Joan W. Scott and Louise Tilly have gone too far in arguing that the work experience of European women was in no way emancipating.[81] French male and female workers proved to be remarkably innovative when faced with the social and economic pressures of the nineteenth century. It is likely that those working-class husbands who supported their wives' decision to abort did so for the same reason they accepted the putting out of their babies to nurse in the country — so as not to lose the wife's contribution to the family income or her participation in the small family enterprise so characteristic of French capitalism.[82] Finally, a study of abortion demonstrates the important role women played in the regulation of family size and casts light on the surge of domestic feminism that marked nineteenth-century France. The recourse of French women to medical self-help reflected an individualism which fits in well with certain models of French behavior such as the Hoffman-Pitts theory of the "delinquent community" and Wylie's discussion of "Systeme D."[83] Few French women bothered with suffrage movements because such associations for positive purposes were not common in France; many simply took matters into their own hands — frequently earlier and more successfully than did women in other countries. In the face of the opposition of the medical, religious and legal professions, they set out to play an active role, by whatever means, to control their fertility. The stress on domestic feminism should not be taken to imply, however, that those concerned with more orthodox feminist causes were indifferent to the subject of fertility control. Madeleine Pelletier's contribution to the abortion discussion has been touched on. To put her activities in context the following chapter provides a full examination of nineteenth-century French feminist attitudes toward restriction of family size.

CHAPTER TEN

Feminism and the Decline of Fertility in France, 1800–1914

In the summer of 1900 the American anarchist-feminist Emma Goldman attended a neo-Malthusian conference in Paris. There she met Paul Robin, the leading French birth control advocate, and was introduced to a variety of contraceptive techniques unknown to her in the United States. Such knowledge she regarded to be of immense importance. Working as a midwife in the slums of New York, Goldman had been repeatedly beseeched by women seeking an end to unwanted pregnancies. "I thought of my former patients on the East Side," she later wrote, "and the blessing it would have meant to them if they could have procured the contraceptives described at these sessions."[1] Goldman's statement raises the question of whether the drop in the French birth rate, which occurred long before similar declines in other western countries, can be taken as evidence of French women enjoying a power not shared by their sisters abroad. Was the restriction of family size a manifestation of a form of domestic feminism? Such claims were certainly advanced by the opponents of such practices. As early as 1782 Père Féline attributed the restriction of the number of children to the concern of husbands to spare their wives the pains of childbirth, and in 1840 Bishop Bouvier similarly linked the small family to women's success in impressing upon men the importance of their wives' health and well-being.[2] By the 1890s this decline in the birth rate was being attributed by a variety of social observers specifically to feminism. According to the eugenicist G. Vacher de Lapouge, evolution was being turned backwards because the finest women were spurning maternity. In a work published in 1896 he declared, "It is a very serious fact that the most intelligent women make the best of their abilities and longer education to provide independent positions for themselves and live celibate lives. This selection poses a danger for the future."[3] In the same year the economist Paul Leroy-Beaulieu noted the relationship between feminism and the fall in natality that had been remarked upon particularly in Anglo-Saxon countries. Such a reciprocal effect was, he asserted, a danger to the state and civilization as a whole because it resulted in the production of smaller, "effeminate" families in which too great attention was poured out by the mother on her one or two children.[4] Political concerns were voiced by Georges Rossignol in yet another study of 1896 in which he declared that women's flouting of natural laws made them potential political radicals. Reversing the reactionary Charles Maurras's statement "I have never seen anarchist mothers and I believe that there are none," Rossignol argued that a wife who spurned childbearing stood a good chance of becoming both a fanatic and an adulteress.[5] The church also had its word to say on feminism. In 1901 Abbé Ract stated that France was falling behind in the population race because the nation was in thrall to the women's movement. Each time the sex roles were upset disorder followed; Ract cited as proof the cruelty of Sparta which was due to its overpowerful women. Ract's curious book also carried a fantastic illustration of a woman dreaming of all the sad, little children she had prevented from being born and hence from reaching paradise; they would forever reproach her for their eternal unhappiness.[6] Approaching the issue from a more down-to-earth angle, Jacques Lux attributed the new desire for "la liberation de la maternité" to the wave of feminism associated with the works of writers such as Ellen Key and Léon Blum. In the 1909 Parliamentary debate Gauthier de Clagny followed the same tack in lashing out at those who "go as far as the extreme limit of the paradox in sustaining this thesis that the woman is mistress of her body."[7] Etienne Lamy of the Académie française shared the view that women had been led astray by those who inculcated the "fear of the child" and claimed that sterility was a "right."

> It was especially the naturally maternal heart of the woman that had to be conquered. One caused her to revolt against the ordeals of pregnancies and the pains of childbearing. One humiliated her by the contempt shown to the gaucheness of motherhood. One taught her that she was mistress of her body, one taught her to be neither chaste nor fertile.[8]

Most of the writers cited above concluded that feminism had to be combatted by providing women with a new education that would stress their duty to reproduce. Dr. J.A. Doléris and Jean Bouscatel in *Néo-malthusianisme: maternité et feminisme: éducation sexuelle* (1918) drew together the threads of such arguments in stating that women had to be taught that they were not free; rather, they had to see themselves as debtors — the married woman in particular as the "irresolvable debtor of society" — until and unless they bore sufficient children.[9]

The statements of these misogynists were frequently bizarre and contradictory but they all centered on the commonplace assumption that the emergence of the French woman's movement and the fall in fertility were related. It seems logical enough to assume that women would have a vital interest in controlling fertility — the previous chapter on abortion should have made that abundantly clear — but the difficulty arises in trying to establish a clear connection between the practice of birth control and the ideology known as feminism. Though France produced a remarkable number of liberated women — one thinks immediately of Mme. de Staël, George Sand, Flora Tristan, Louise Michel — French feminism was not as powerful and united a movement as that of the Anglo-Saxon countries. Why was this? A variety of hypotheses can be advanced. It could be that feminists in France were plagued by the inability — a failing that Stanley Hoffman asserts is common to the French in general — to organize for positive purposes.[10] A nation of critics does not produce the kind of citizens attracted to constructive organizations. Also, the Protestant nations, in leaving charity activities to women, may have unwittingly offered them avenues such as the temperance campaigns and the philanthropic movements by which they could apprentice themselves in political activity. In Catholic France, however, such opportunities were limited because the male members of the church and state continued to predominate in such affairs. The fact that nineteenth-century French feminism was usually associated with socialism because of the interest taken in it by men such as Saint-Simon, Enfantin, Fourier, Considerant, and Leroux could also have prevented feminism from having had a broader appeal. Indeed, even in the twentieth century the French feminists continued to be divided into conservative and socialist factions. But the problem with all these hypotheses is that they take the English and American feminist movements as models in contrast to which the French experience cannot avoid appearing immature. In particular these arguments fail to relate French feminism to the most dramatic aspects of French women's lives in the nineteenth century — the fact that France's birth rate was the lowest in the western world and that the percentage of women in the active work force was the highest.

　　Little has been written concerning the relationship between French feminism and the decline in family size, but John and Olive Banks have argued in *Feminism and Family Planning* that in England there is no evidence of any such link. English feminists, assert the Banks, focused their attention solely on the question of the franchise and purposefully shunned the issue of birth control for fear that it might compromise their political program.[11] The Banks conclude that when the English birth rate dropped it was due not to the success of feminist arguments, but to decisions made by men based on economic calculation. How does the French situation compare to the English? Given that fertility fell much earlier in France than in England although the French feminist movement was weaker and more divided, it could be argued that the Banks' hypothesis is amply confirmed. But at least one student of French feminism, while asserting that nineteenth-century French feminists "never advocated birth control," comes to conclusions almost totally opposed to those of the Banks — that French feminists did not have to defend birth control because it was already so widely practiced.[12]

Both of the above interpretations are simplistic inasmuch as they rely on the notion of a monolithic entity known as "feminism" defined in a narrowly political sense that automatically excludes almost every female advocate of fertility control. There were French feminists who were opposed to birth control on moral grounds just as there were others who felt no need to mention what they regarded to be a common private practice, but there was also a third group in whose writings can be found a current of thought linking feminism and fertility. An analysis of their works reveals how in making maternity a question of crucial importance the feminists of the 1830s laid the basis for the argument advanced by their counterparts of the 1890s — that motherhood could only be freely and consciously entered into by controlling fertility. Far from being uninterested in the problems posed by childbearing, these French feminists as women were quite naturally preoccupied by them. The solutions they proposed — abstinence or free love, maternity benefits or birth control — which on the surface appeared so disparate, all reflected the same appreciation for the necessity of turning the powers of fertility to serve the purposes of women.

At first glance the first generation of French feminists hardly seems a group in which one would have any chance of finding the origins of an interest in birth control. Responding to the espousal of Malthusian theories by some women in England, Désirée Gay declared in 1848:

> As women . . . we protest the ideas of Malthus. We have witnessed with pain, these past few years, the activities of Miss Martineau and several other intelligent English women who have declared themselves in favor of a doctrine . . . that is immoral.[13]

What has to be recalled, however, is that the "immorality" which Malthus recommended consisted of postponement of marriage, not employment of contraceptives. The early feminists such as Gay, Suzanne Voilquin, Claire Démar, and Pauline Roland attacked such suggestions because they construed them as an attack upon women's power of maternity.[14] The first step in advancing the claims of women's emancipation was taken not surprisingly along the path already laid out by Rousseau in the eighteenth century and Claire de Rémusat, Pauline Guizot, and Albertine Necker de

Saussure in the nineteenth, which led to an exalting of woman's childbearing role. What the early feminists attempted to do was to turn the accepted importance of maternity into an argument for women's greater freedom. Maternity was therefore lauded and defended in a quasi-religious Saint-Simonian language. In Suzanne Voilquin's words:

> But maternity! It is our most beautiful attribute; it encompasses all other feelings without excluding a one, it is woman in her full flowering. In the religion of the future it will no longer be a virginal madonna, as a feminine model that we will present for the adoration of the Believers: it will be the mother![15]

In seeking greater esteem for women's functions these early feminists claimed that women's reproductive power gave them the right to demand equality with men, who had access only to productive power. Voilquin in the preface to Démar's *Ma loi d'avenir* (1834) proclaimed:

> To you men *production*, the great works of clearing, the conquest of the land, of the material world. To us *population*, to us to renew humanity, to us it belongs to form the hearts, the sentiments of man, to us finally the moral education of the world.[16]

And in similar language Gay wrote in 1848:

> A great social reform is necessary, inevitable, but this reform, in order to be complete and durable cannot emanate from man alone. Man only knows how to establish order through despotism, woman only knows how to organize by the strength of her motherly love. But together they will know how to gain order and freedom.[17]

Much of this sounds quite conservative. In fact the feminists such as Démar and Roland associated with the *Tribune des femmes* were to employ the Saint-Simonian notions of different but complementary sex roles for the radical purpose of freeing maternity from male domination. Thus following the praise of maternity came the attack on paternity, "le pouvoir monstreux," as Démar described it. Roland posited the idea of the necessity of a new society in which the mother would no longer have to be dependent upon the male. Indeed, Roland herself ran the risk of unwed motherhood.

> I want to become a mother, but with paternity unknown. I have questioned myself severely on this subject. I asked myself whether, in the sick state that pregnancy always brings on, I would be strong enough not to ask a man to give a name to the child in the eyes of the world, to whom he would be father before God. I also asked myself whether I had the right to bring into the world a being who would be rejected because

of his birth. I resolved both questions affirmatively: I will be proud of my maternity and my child will be proud of his birth.[18]

Démar went so far as to even denigrate childrearing after having lauded childbearing:

No more motherhood; . . . Woman must work, fulfill a function; and how can she, if she is always condemned to fill a more or less long part of her life by attending to the education of one or more children. Either the work will be neglected or poorly done, or the child will be poorly brought up, deprived of the care that his weakness and his lengthy period of growth demand.[19]

Thus what can be detected in the writings of those feminists of the first half of the nineteenth century who were associated with utopian socialists such as Saint-Simon and Fourier is not a simple enthusiasm for mindless reproduction. Flora Tristan expressed her shock that any women should be subjected to such a fate. "Alas! she is reduced to the position of a child-making machine."[20] Rather, these feminists were elaborating the argument that childbearing was so important that it could not be undertaken casually. Moreover, the function was so vital to women's status and well-being that it could not be, asserted the early propagandists, subjected to male domination.

The early feminist argument did not advance much beyond an exaltation of maternity, and the charged, mystical language in which much of it was couched read rather strangely once the utopian expectations of the Fourierists and Saint-Simonians died away at mid-century. Nevertheless, these early works provided the basis for the future argument of what was to be known as "la maternité consciente."

France experienced its second surge of feminist activity in the 1860s, focusing for the most part on responses to the misogynist musings of Proudhon and Michelet. In the writings of Juliette Lamber, André Léo, and Jenny P. d'Hericourt the focus of feminine attention shifted from the question of maternity to women's work, just as the language in which the arguments were expressed became less romantic and more commonsensical.[21] In part this transition reflected social changes. Women represented 28 percent of the active population in 1866, 30 percent in 1872, 38.9 percent in 1906. As women worked more and more outside the home, the ideal of female beauty changed "as Zola observed, from the plump, large thighed, heavy-breasted mother to a more boyish, sylphlike form."[22] The feminist transition also reflected the concern that males were seeking to make maternity a gilded cage from which no escape was possible. André Léo in *La Femme et les moeurs* (1869) declared that Proudhon and Michelet were equally insulting in applauding maternity while hypocritically asserting that women were inferior.[23] Jenny P. d'Hericourt in *La Femme affranchie* (1860) added Comte to the list of woman-haters, and charged them all with seeking to use appeals to love to counter women's demands for reason and justice.[24] Juliette Lamber attacked the most famous misogynist of the nineteenth century head-on in *Idées anti-proudhoniennes.* (1860). She set aside Proudhon's claim that the only purpose of love was reproduction as "too old-fashioned, too out of keeping with universal thinking to have any power of proselytism on our contemporaries." The maternal role was, of course, of central importance, but women could not, argued Lamber, be restricted to this one function.

> I maintain that it is not true that family life is adequate for the physical, moral, and intellectual activity of woman. The role of mother hen is doubtlessly very respectable but it does not suit everyone and is not as engrossing as it is said to be.[25]

Women would continue to be wives and mothers but their emancipation depended upon access to employment.

The second generation of feminists, like the first, said nothing directly about the artificial restriction of fertility. They did, however, produce a more nuanced picture of maternity by warding off the arguments of those who, like Proudhon and Michelet, employed appeals to love and motherhood to restrict women's options. The importance placed on motherhood by the early feminists was not disavowed, but the tacit assumption which underlay much of the writing on women's right to work was that freedom from unwanted pregnancies was possible and desirable.

Both the organized feminist movement and the birth control movement emerged in France at the end of the nineteenth century. They are usually treated in isolation but each expressed in its own way a response to common problems faced by French women. Paul Robin was a feminist of long standing as demonstrated by his defense in the International Working Men's Association of women's right to work and his pioneering activities in coeducation. His interest in birth control was similarly based on the conviction that it provided the only sure basis for full female emancipation. In *Aux gens mariés*, one of his first tracts, he defended the argument first sketched out by the early feminists that the woman had a right "to be a mother only when she has decided, after full consideration. It is the first step, the most essential point of the real emancipation of the woman, and as a consequence of the whole race."[26] And Robin further asserted that the first priority of any contraceptive technique was that it be fully controlled by the woman.

From the beginning of his birth control activities Robin sought to recruit women activists to the cause because he believed that only they could counter the fatalism of wives who put up with repeated unwanted pregnancies. Working-class women in particular needed to be told there was a way out. The letter of a young woman of the Bastille *quartier* was reprinted in *Régénération* describing her husband's uncontrolled sexual demands.[27] Robin was aware that many sexual encounters in poor households were marked by both ignorance and brutality. It was his belief that such incidents could be avoided only if women engaged themselves more actively in the birth control campaign.[28] For too long the discussion had been monopolized by men. Indeed, some women were becoming obviously restive, for when Frédéric Passy attacked Robin's population views in 1897 at the Société d'économie politique a woman in the audience cried out, "They speak about women at the fireside just as they would speak of the dog in its kennel."[29]

The 1890s witnessed the emergence of a number of women who, in part responding to the challenge laid down by Robin, publicly asserted the necessary relationship of birth control to female emancipation. These women, coming from a variety of backgrounds and political persuasions, ranged from individual eccentrics such as Marie Huot, to bourgeois journalists such as Marguerite Durand, to radical doctors such as Madeleine Pelletier. On the rare occasions when the activities of these women have been noted they have been taken out of the context of nineteenth-century French feminism. Certainly, they were not part of the conservative mainstream at the turn of the century, but their ideas can only be fully understood if seen as part of an evolving appreciation, begun in the 1830s and climaxing in the 1890s, of the concept of "maternité consciente." What united all these activists was the belief that the primary importance of birth control lay not in its social, economic, or demographic effects but in the power it offered women to control their own lives.

The first and in many ways the most curious feminist defender of birth control was Marie Huot.[30] Indeed, her public discussion of contraception predated Robin's lectures. In September of 1892 in the rooms of the Société de géographie on the boulevard Saint-Germain, Huot voiced what was to become the notorious slogan of women's revolt, the "grève de ventre." It would be a gross simplification to describe Huot as merely a birth controller and feminist. Her greatest fame sprang from her earlier defense not of women, but of animals. The two interests, however, were not that far apart in the nineteenth century, and in both England and France the antivivisection movement brought together many women hostile to male medical scientists subjecting any being to needless pain.[31] In England the birth controller Annie Besant was converted to antivivisection by Maria Kingsford; Huot, who was a great admirer of Kingsford and Besant, appears to have moved in the opposite direction, from antivivisection to birth control. In the early 1890s Huot was the force behind the Ligue populaire contre la vivisection and gained notoriety by her umbrella attack upon the anatomist C.E. Brown-Séquard. Accordingly, in 1892 when she broached the tabooed subject of fertility control, she had a large audience, reported in the press as close to two thousand.[32] Like earlier feminists she attacked Proudhon for seeking to limit woman to the roles of wife and mother, but she went on to ask why a radical like Louise Michel would call for larger working-class families when so many were struck down by illness and poverty. Women had to restrict their fertility. The bourgeoisie were already employing such practices, but these *cafards paillards* were keeping the necessary information from the proletariat. Huot was herself not terribly forthcoming when it came to specifics and did not respond to the audience's cries of "Indiquez-nous des remèdes, des moyens." She did, however, imply that she did not believe that abortion should be considered a crime.

Huot gave the first public lecture in France on the necessity of birth control but it was also to be her last on the topic. Though continuing to follow the population debate, the "mère aux chats," as she was known, was apparently too taken up by her other interests to make any further contributions.[33] The importance of Huot's talk was that it placed birth control clearly on the feminist and socialist agendas. A few anarchist students in the audience had responded to such an idea with the chant "Conspuez Malthus, conspuez," but Huot retorted that the emancipation of the woman and the working class as a whole could only be gained by the "grève de ventre."

By the turn of the century more comprehensive feminist examinations of fertility control began to appear in the women's press. Marguerite Durand, a wealthy bourgeois feminist, and editor of the all-woman paper *La Fronde*, supported Robin's Ligue and opened her journal's columns to a discussion of his proposals. In 1898 Mme. de Bouet contributed an article attacking the anti-Malthusians and asked why those parading their concern for France's depopulation produced such small families. Jane Saulnier moved more directly to the heart of the matter in asserting that maternity was the key to feminism. For some, motherhood was woman's highest calling; for others a mere animal function. In either case maternity could only be turned to woman's advantage if it were made a conscious act. In 1903 *La Fronde* carried a full debate of the concept of "maternité consciente"; some claimed that it was criminal to have large families but others such as Ida R. Sée argued that woman's freedom would not be extended if she were restricted to a certain number of pregnancies. *La Fronde* did not limit itself simply to the question of contraception; even the issue of abortion was broached by Jeanne H. Caruchet, who defended that act as a form of protest by the woman who was "l'esclave de ses organes, après avoir été souvent, celle de l'homme."[34]

Better known than *La Fronde* as a mouthpiece for birth control propaganda was the left-wing paper *La femme affranchie* under the editorship of Gabrielle Petit. In its columns feminism, socialism, antimilitarism and neo-Malthusianism were combined to produce a heady brew. Petit elaborated a defense of birth control that put the greatest stress on the duty of women to spare themselves and their children the pain and misery that often resulted from additional unwanted pregnancies. Petit preached this message not only in the columns of her paper, but also via leaflets and in public talks as well.[35]

Durand and Petit were both sympathetic to the birth control cause and gave it a fair hearing in their papers; in the case of Nelly Roussel and Madeleine Pelletier one finally comes to two feminists who were totally devoted to the campaign, for they regarded it not as complementary but as essential to women's emancipation. Roussel wrote for the birth control publications *Régénération* and *Nouvelle régénération* as well as for a string of radical papers including *Action* and the *Almanach feministe*.[36]

According to Roussel, feminism was necessary to break old cultural constraints and permit women to become "real" women. But in turn this required that feminists support the notion of "la maternité consciente" by defending the woman's freedom to select the moment of conception, by asserting the right of every woman to motherhood, and by demanding "le juste salaire du noble travail maternel."[37] In Roussel's argument one can hear the echoes of the sentiments first expressed by the Saint-Simonian feminists. Like them Roussel demanded that maternity be recognized as a social function and accordingly be supported by the state. From this it followed that Roussel could downplay the importance of the "recherche de la paternité"; it was more important to allow women and children to do without men than to attempt to extort from males a paltry maintenance. But Roussel went beyond the early feminists in adding that a woman's full freedom could only be attained if protection from conception were possible. Restriction of fertility represented a form of "revolt" against the dictates of nature and the dominance of men.[38] The fact that some feminists refused to defend birth control Roussel attributed to timidity. Some of them perhaps had been dissuaded by the hostility of doctors toward birth control, but Roussel caustically suggested that asking medical men their advice on such practices was akin to asking brewers for their views on the temperance movement. And of those women dissuaded by the hostility of socialists toward birth control Roussel asked if it were not true that the left "speaks of revolution always and thinks of it never," consistently denigrating middle-class women? In short, Roussel argued that it was up to women to seize their own freedom, and only birth control could make such an emancipation complete.

Many of the same arguments expressed in a more vehement tone were advanced by the remarkable Dr. Madeleine Pelletier. Having already fought many battles to win places in two male preserves — the Socialist Party and the medical profession — Pelletier thought nothing of jeopardizing her position by moving on to defend both contraception and abortion.[39] She castigated socialist women through her paper *La Suffragiste* for not supporting feminism, and she castigated feminists in her tracts for not supporting birth control. According to Pelletier, the existing society was one in which women were little more than "bêtes de travail, bêtes d'amour" subject to men. Women were used by males for their sexual pleasure, but female needs and desires went without recognition. Pelletier's utopia, like that of the Saint-Simonian feminists, would be one in which free love and matriarchy existed and where women could raise their children without the assistance of men. But in the existing society such dreams of independence were crushed by the burdens of pregnancy that plunged back into subjection even the most intellectually liberated woman. Were childrearing collectivized, were women economically self-sufficient, pregnancy would be a joy, but in the existing state all one could hope to do was provide women with contraceptive information and, if that proved insufficient, recourse to abortion. Practicing what she preached, Pelletier provided abortions for needy women and ended her life incarcerated because of her activities.[40]

This current of thought in French feminism, which ironically began by exalting maternity and ended in calling for its conscious restriction, was by no means the dominant element in the woman's movement. By the 1870s one could speak of a "movement" rather than of clusters of feminist thinkers: the Association for the Rights of Women had emerged under the leadership of Léon Richer and Maria Desraimes. The movement had limited goals, simply the attainment of legal equality for women, and was marked by republicanism and anticlericalism.[41] Indeed, it was not until the late 1870s that Hubertine Auclert raised the issue of women's suffrage. The relative conservatism of the movement was in part due to the fact that it was organized in the decade following the Commune when the left was in disarray. Moreover, Richer and Desraimes sought to defuse opposition to feminism by arguing that it would strengthen rather than undermine the social fabric of the republic. Accordingly, the goals of the movement were restricted well into the twentieth century to women's admission to education, the abolition of the civil incapacities of married women, the reform of laws relating to property and authority over children, the establishment of divorce, the end to legalized prostitution, and the legitimation of paternity suits. The questions of sexual liberation raised by the Saint-Simonian feminists were dropped and only resurfaced in the writings of those interested in fertility control. Consequently, at the beginning of the twentieth century there was on one side a small group of feminist radicals who placed great stress on the question of sexuality, and on the other the larger number of conservative feminists who avoided the issue. The most important feminist organization, the Conseil national des femmes françaises, not only restricted its activities to the campaign for the vote; to prove its moral rectitude in 1909 it demanded the creation of an organization to *oppose* birth control.[42] As a result in 1911 the Ligue contre le crime d'avortement was formed. The sentiments of the conservative faction were summed up by Auclert, who asserted: "Maternity will cease to terrify French women when, instead of dishonoring or reducing them to dependency, it [France] honors them by payments for indispensable service to the state."[43] Interestingly, many of the socialist feminists expressed much the same sentiments. Feminists within the socialist movement were more or less reduced to the level of a woman's auxiliary. Some no doubt favored birth control, but because the leadership equated such practices with Malthusian economic arguments, the socialist feminists had to follow the party line of opposition to family restriction.[44] The French experience was not unique. In Germany, for example, Zetkin, Luxemburg, and Braun were not certain if contraception and abortion were immoral, but they concluded that they could not in any case be given serious consideration. Even if these practices did benefit individuals their defense by the party could jeopardize its electoral success.[45] The same line was followed in France. The leading feminist within the French Socialist Party, Aline Valette, assumed the responsibility of attacking the proponents of birth control. She argued that the degenerate social state in which abortion and contraception flourished would pass with the victory of socialism. Fertility was declining as a result of capitalism; after the Revolution women could return to their natural roles and fertility would rise: "If women today seem to evade their primary purpose, maternity, it is in order to return to it more surely, with independence, serenity, and dignity assured."[46]

The fact that all feminists did not rally to the support of birth control naturally disappointed Paul Robin. In 1896, in addressing an international feminist congress in Paris, he lamented the fact that some radical feminists, including the daughters of Elisée Reclus, were proclaiming their belief in "libre amour" as a sort of "propaganda par le fait" against patriarchal society. Robin's response was that free love only worked if the woman had not the "right" — Robin declared it an absurd word — but the knowledge and means of controlling fertility.[47] Why then did not more feminists openly support the birth control campaign? One reason that Robin apparently overlooked was that they did not relish the thought of again following the dictates of a man. Robin did not make matters any better in setting himself up as the arbiter of "vrai feminime." He declared, "Le mot 'feminisme' est un mot de bataille evidement antihommiste," and lectured women on the need to recognize the fact that their *only* problem was that posed by childbearing.[48] Even a female birth controller such as Gabrielle Petit likely antagonized potential recruits in cruelly referring to the mothers of large families as "ces nonchalantes," "ces ignorantes," the "pauvres lâches" who committed the "crime" of bearing unwanted children.[49]

Not as many feminists defended birth control as Robin would have wished, but this should not blind us to the fact that in France women were far more candid in discussing the issue than in either England or America.[50] The fact that from the 1830s on a current of feminism highlighted the importance of maternity provided the basis for the final argument of the importance of controlling fertility. Moreover, the overwhelming evidence that millions of ordinary French women were already seeking to regulate their reproduction goaded the conscientious into providing a public apology for private practices. France at the turn of the century was known as a country in which the women not only controlled their fertility but proclaimed their right to do so. This chapter began with an account of Emma Goldman's visit to France in 1900. Thirteen years later Margaret Sanger, who was to become the moving force behind the American birth control movement, made the same pilgrimage and expressed the same surprise about the sophisticated knowledge of French women.

> When Bill Haywood began taking me into the homes of the syndi-
> calists, I found perfect acceptance of family limitation and its relation to
> labor.
> "Have you just discovered this?" I asked each woman I met.
> "Oh no, *Maman* told me."
> "Well, who told her?"
> "*Grandmère*, I suppose" . . .
> Some of the contraceptive formulas which have been handed
> down were almost as good as those of today. Although they had to
> make simple things, mothers prided themselves on their special recipes
> for suppositories as much as on those for *pot au feu* or wine. All
> individual Frenchwomen consider this knowledge their individual right,
> and, if it failed, abortion, which was still common. I talked about the
> problems of my own people, but they could give me no help, merely
> shrugging their shoulders, apparently glad they were living in France and
> not in the United States.[51]

PART FIVE

The Backlash

CHAPTER ELEVEN

Depopulation and Degeneration

Was the birth control campaign waged by Robin, Humbert, Pelletier, and Roussel of real importance in the decline of French fertility? The best argument that can be advanced to support its significance is based on the fact that following the First World War the French government passed harsh laws against such activities as part of its pronatalist crusade. This study began by noting the passage by the French Chamber in 1920 of statutes outlawing the distribution of contraceptive information and tightening up the laws on abortion. In part these bills were a direct response to the enormous losses in French manpower resulting from the war. Fifteen percent of all men between the ages of eighteen and forty-eight — one million three hundred thousand in all — had been killed and another three million wounded. Not only had the mortality rate risen during the war; the birth rate had precipitously declined. The number of marriages was cut by three-fourths in the first year of the war, though it leaped up again at its end and was followed by a minor baby boom. In fact the loss in births between 1914 and 1918 was never made up. The birth rate dropped from 18.2 per thousand in 1913 to 9.5 per thousand in 1916. Once the system of leaves for the troops was established, which permitted men to return periodically from the front, natality picked up; in 1918 it reached 12.2 per thousand and stood at 12.6 per thousand in 1919, but in total approximately one million seven hundred thousand babies, which if the birth rate of 1913 had been sustained would have been born, failed to appear.[1]

The deputies of the rightist Bloc National that dominated the 1919 assembly — called the "Chambre bleu horizon" because so many of its members had only recently returned from the front — were naturally inclined to support drastic measures deemed appropriate in light of the country's population losses. But to appreciate fully the forces behind the passage of the antibirth-control legislation it is necessary to see it as the culmination of the long struggle of populationists launched in the 1870s against the forces of depopulation. The defeat suffered in 1871 at the hands of Prussia initiated a half century of French demographic discussion that finally climaxed in the laws passed after the victory of 1918. Each decade witnessed the rekindling of the fear of French depopulation, exacerbated by the menace of German growth. The obvious spur to such concerns was that the decline in fertility was viewed not primarily as a moral problem, but as a political danger in that it weakened France at home, limited her diplomatic options abroad, and encouraged the adoption by Germany of an adventurist foreign policy. The loudest of the opening salvos in the populationist campaign was fired by Alfred Pernessin writing as "Dr. Rommel" in *Au pays de la revanche* (1886). The great effectiveness of this work lay in the rage it engendered in the nationalist reading public by the gloating of a supposed foreigner over the nation's weaknesses. Rommel attributed the decline in French natality to the general decadence of society symbolized by political corruption, overcentralization, increased taxation, growing bureaucratization, and the accompanying alienation of the masses. The country was portrayed as being economically weak and hiding behind its tariffs; its citizens as insecure and seeking to achieve security by limiting the size of their families. The peasant had a small family because he feared having to divide his land; the bourgeois adopted the same tactic to avoid "des tracas, des ennuis, de la gêne."[2] Rommel concluded, in terms tailored to raise the hackles of conservatives, that France, having given evidence of its timidity, would have to make way for its more vigorous and populous neighbors.

Rommel's provocative work was meant to frighten its readers by raising the specter of an inevitably expanding Germany; his premises were not, however, accepted by all. There were still some vocal defenders of laissez-faire attitudes toward population in the 1880s. Jean Boillot, for example, responded to Rommel by asserting proudly that France's low fertility was not due to lack of vigor or potency; rather, it had to be seen as a sign of prudence and rationality. Such growth might be slow but it was regular, and as a result the French did not have to seek, like the Germans, outlets for overpopulation in emigration. France's small families were a manifestation of a mature, civilized culture which, Boillot confidently claimed, was clearly preferable to this "fever of procreation which has possessed the Germans and this fever of industry which dazzles them."[3] But by the 1890s such scoffing at the development of the industrializing power across the Rhine was heard with declining frequency. Georges Rossignol, writing as "Roger Debury" in a study of 1896, echoed Rommel's warnings in lamenting the decline in willpower underlying the fall in fertility. The "duty" to provide children for the defense of the republic was being increasingly shirked by women unprepared for motherhood.[4] This same stress on duty was made by Fernand Boverat in *Patriotisme et paternité*, which appeared a year before the outbreak of the First World War. After a somewhat awkward introduction in which he attempted to answer in advance critics who might make the charge that

Boverat, having no children himself, was hardly one to pontificate on the subject of paternity, he launched into an assault on those who ignored the fact that France was already "at war" with Germany. This war, he asserted, was being lost as a result of birth control. The neo-Malthusian propaganda in circulation for nearly thirty years he held responsible for depriving France of approximately 250,000 births a year.[5]

In such sensationalist accounts of France's population problem the birth controllers always received their share of abuse, but the degree of culpability attributed to them varied according to the individual author's interpretation of events. The most pessimistic critics accepted the notion that the decline in fertility was at least due in part to involuntary causes. Gustave Le Bon and Georges Vacher de Lapouge argued that mass impotence was a result of the decadence of morals. Lapouge in particular linked the phenomenon to what he saw as racial deterioration, and to support his argument he sought to relate natality to a cephalic index. As France's last Aryan bastions in Brittany, the Jura, the Vosges, and the Pyrenees, fell as a result of intermarriage, so too would the birth rate. In such a schema the activity of birth control propagandists was presumably of little importance but they still bore a portion of guilt. Because of the availability of such information, women were now avoiding what was in Lapouge's eyes their natural condition — either being pregnant or lactating. Instead, they were menstruating, the ovaries were overworked, and the resulting hereditary disease of "ovarites" further reduced fecundity.[6] Similar, though less imaginative, interpretations that linked diseases and sterility were advanced by Picon, Maurel, and Félice. They pointed to tuberculosis, venereal disease, alcoholism, obesity, and overuse of tobacco as playing contributing roles.[7]

These physiological explanations of France's fertility decline were countered by Catholic apologists who claimed that it was loss of faith, not any fall in virility, that was responsible for France's woes. In chapter two the church's position was analyzed and there is no need to review its arguments at length here. It is worth noting, however, the way in which the population issue was used by both Catholics and their opponents to lash out at each other. Priests such as Ract held doctors and scientists accountable for popularizing materialistic doctrines that justified contraception, while eugenicists like Lapouge accused the church of undercutting fertility by its effeminate doctrines.[8] A compromise solution was offered by the positivist Georges Deherme, who accepted Lapouge's contention that at the moment only the unfit multiplied but argued that the situation could be reversed if a "positivist religion" were preached.[9]

Both the physiological and the religious arguments related the restriction of fertility to some vaguely defined "evil" of physical or psychological origin so deeply rooted that the chances of eradicating it appeared remote. The interpretations offered by academic sociologists and demographers were far less pathologically oriented. They tended in the main to assume that the restriction of births was volitional, not involuntary, and therefore hope was held out that the population growth could be manipulated by the government's adoption of the right sort of policies. For classical liberals, of course, the less government the better. Old Malthusians like Frédéric Passy opposed state intervention on principle and argued that the government had no right in penalizing people who decided to have small families.[10] Some Malthusians changed their stripes. Paul Robin was shocked to discover that Yves Guyot, once an enthusiastic defender of Malthusian economics, was by the mid-1890s condemning the "suicide of families."[11] Those who kept the liberal faith but shared the concern for France's falling fertility found a way out of their predicament by declaring that the problem was caused, and consequently could not be cured, by government encroachments. It was fiscal interference, tariff protection, child labor legislation, and government centralization that they pointed to as the curbs on fertility.[12]

Liberal economists focused on the individual; Frédéric Le Play and his followers were preoccupied by the family. Although his death in 1885 occurred before the depopulation scare had climaxed, Le Play had sketched out in his works the argument that restriction of fertility was a sign of family instability. In turn he attributed this instability to the French Revolution, which had been responsible for forcing peasants to provide their heirs with equal portions. The loss of testamentary freedom resulted in farmers' preferring to have only one son to whom they could pass on their land intact, rather than seeing it divided into unprofitable sections among a host of offspring. Le Play's theory did not explain why the birth rate varied from département to département; it obviously did not apply to landless urban workers, but it did appeal to conservatives who assumed France's demographic difficulties had to be related to the decline of the patriarchal family. Le Play's disciples formed La Reforme sociale to fight for the reestablishment of testamentary freedom and the decentralization of government. Only by returning power to the father, they asserted, could the unstable, "nomadic" existence of families, so deleterious in effect on population growth, be ended.[13] The forces of custom having been undermined by political and industrial revolution, it was necessary for the hierarchy to institute new restraints to guarantee social peace. The sign of the success of a family system was, claimed Le Play, its fertility; judged by this standard, the nuclear household had obviously failed.

Le Play's followers tended to be conservative; those of Arsène Dumont, socialist. Dumont, the best known population theorist at the turn of the century, undertook his investigations with the vow that if they did not result in getting him the professorship in the School of Anthropology as a reward, he would commit suicide. He did not get it and he killed himself. Dumont's fame, however, rested on his elaboration of the concept of "social capillarity" as an explanation for France's falling birth rate. He posited there could exist no desire to advance in a society in which there was no possibility of mobility. Consequently, large families would not be a burden. In a democracy, however, citizens were given political equality and had dangled before them opportunities for social and economic improvement that could only be seized by the sacrifice of fertility. It followed, then, that the resigned were fecund while the ambitious were sterile. Beginning from socialist and antireligious premises, Dumont elaborated a population theory that was also a critique of existing society, inasmuch as he saw it as one in which the development of the individual could only be in inverse proportion to the development of the race.[14] In response to Robin's argument that contraception could be employed to improve society, he replied that neo-Malthusians were unpatriotic and unscientific. Regarding the low rate of population growth, he declared himself shocked that "there is one Frenchman who is pleased by it, who wishes it to be made worse, and recommends surgical means capable of procuring abortion and lowering natality."[15] In Dumont's work there was an echo of the old mercantilist doctrine that prosperity and culture depended on population density, but it was also colored by new social-psychological concerns such as Durkheim's that suicides were more frequent in small families, where collective sentiments were not as strong, than in larger families.[16] Though politically far removed from Le Play, Dumont came to somewhat similar conclusions. For the health of the nation to be restored the rights of the collectivity had to be reasserted over those of the individual.

Paul Leroy-Beaulieu, the last of the main demographic theorists writing before the First World War, did not share such pessimistic beliefs. In general he followed Herbert Spencer and H. Carey in linking the fall in natality to the rise of civilization. If France's growth had been curbed at an early date it was only because it had been introduced by the Revolution to a calculating, rational world into which all nations would eventually enter. That the neo-Malthusians were a manifestation of such an evolution Leroy-Beaulieu was willing to admit. Indeed, he confessed that when still a young man he had been given a translation of George Drysdale's *Elements of Social Science*, "by a well-known and well-respected French philanthropist, who presented it to me as the summation of all of social science."[17] But though Leroy-Beaulieu accepted the long-term fall in fertility as inescapable, he also spoke out against symptoms of the evolution which he regarded as unhealthy. He sought to curb the overweening desire of working-class youths to move rapidly up the social scale by adapting the school system to stress vocational training; he labeled a danger to the state the activities of feminists in relating emancipation and the restriction of family size; and he castigated the birth controllers as "a sort of Malthusian church and Malthusian press which celebrates every obstacle, even the most immoral, to fertility."[18]

The general consensus of contributors to the demographic debate was that the decline in fertility was a bad thing. Indeed, the term "depopulation" was frequently employed to suggest that France's population growth was not only slowing down, but also might be ended if the birth rate were overtaken by the death rate. What measures did these observers suggest to meet the crisis? They were of two sorts, both negative and positive measures. The chief negative measure would be the passage of laws against contraception and abortion for the purpose of *preventing* couples from limiting family size. We will return to this issue in a moment. The positive measures consisted of a wide range of proposed reforms that would *encourage* marriage and the bearing and rearing of children.

To have children it is necessary to have couples. The fact that many workers either did not marry or preferred to live in a free union rather than legitimate their relationship was pointed out by many as being detrimental to population growth. It was not so much that the poor did not want to marry; the problem was that they found it difficult to do so. Laws required the consent of parents for sons up to the age of twenty-five and daughters up to twenty-one; the marriage could take place only where residence had been established; and the necessary assemblying of a "dossier matrimonial" involved certain expenses. Domestics and soldiers were two classes of workers who were portrayed as facing special difficulties because of employment far from home. In the first half of the century the Société charitable de Saint François Régis undertook the provision of funds to facilitate marriages of workers already cohabiting. Some of the couples so united had in fact been living together for decades and raised families. Between 1826 and 1869 the Society reported 45,800 such marriages in Paris and an accompanying 28,645 legitimations. In Lyon, 12,292 were wed, in Marseilles 9,844, and in Lille 11,941. Other societies such as that of Saint-Vincent de Paul were also involved in similar activities, and altogether 151,610 *mariages réparateurs* were carried out in the département of the Seine between 1856 and 1867, a figure close to one-ninth of all marriages. The problems faced by the single were only eased by the laws of 20 June 1896 and 21 June 1907, fought for by Abbé Lemire, which lowered the age at which consent of parents was required and reduced residency requirements. In 1909, however, Charles

Lyon-Caen asserted that the expense of registering marriages still posed an obstacle to some.[19]

Populationists wanted easier access to marriage because all information suggested that such unions were more fruitful than common-law arrangements. The former arrangements also provided greater protection for children as indicated by lower infant mortality rates. What preoccupied many was the fact that if a child was born before the marriage of his or her parents it was difficult, if not impossible, for the woman, because of the law forbidding the "recherche de paternité" mentioned in the chapter on abortion, to force the man to accept his responsibilities. This law was presented by populationists as an incitement to seduction and its abrogation called for. Some minor changes were made in the legislation before the First World War, a process slowed by such men as Lucien Cazals, who argued that to remove the law would permit women to foist their illegitimate children on innocent men of substance.[20]

Ironically, one of the arguments used in favor of divorce, reestablished in 1884, was that it too would profit population growth. This line of thought was based on the premise that unhappy marriages would not be fertile and infertile marriages would not be happy. In either case divorce would permit the spouses to separate and find more compatible fertile unions. Catholic opponents of divorce disagreed and responded that both legal separation and birth control were products of a decadent age, each representing in its own way an avoidance of legitimate responsibilities. Henry Joly advanced figures to show that families were smallest where divorce was most employed, but such a finding could hardly be surprising given the fact that the legal expenses limited access to all but the wealthy.[21]

Assuming that a couple did marry, what would prevent it from raising a large family? Economic constraints obviously played a major role. Edme Piot and Colonel G. Toutée called for fiscal reforms to remedy the situation by penalizing bachelors and small families on the one hand, while providing tax relief for large families on the other.[22] An important aspect of the economic burdens facing the large family were exorbitant rents and inadequate housing, topics touched on by Martial and Beaufreton.[23] Unhealthy tenements not only limited the number of children, but they also endangered the children who were born. According to Paul Strauss and Henri de Rothschild, concerned by the lamentably high infant mortality rates, it was just as important to protect the babies already existing as to goad mothers into producing even more.[24]

Would the freedom a father enjoyed in apportioning his wealth among his children further affect his family strategies? Such had been the argument of Le Play and it was carried on by La Réforme sociale. Minor changes were made in the inheritance law in 1894, 1908, and 1909, and the topic continued to preoccupy commentators since so many assumed that France's demographic situation had been created by the peasant's desire to protect his land from divisions. The argument did not go unopposed. Some pointed out that in countries such as Belgium and Holland, where primogeniture had been maintained, the birth rate was also falling. Others argued that the real point in conservatives' supporting a return to testamentary freedom was not so much to increase population growth as to reinforce social inequalities. Colonel Toutée and Gustave Rouanet, for example, called for more, rather than less, state intervention in inheritance matters so that poor, large families would be rewarded and small, wealthy families penalized.[25]

The outburst of populationist propagandizing was given expression in a wide range of institutions. The Académie des sciences morales et politiques studied the issue of depopulation in 1906, as did the École de la science sociale in 1908; discussions were held in Paris in 1910 by the École des hautes études sociales and the Conférence internationale pour la répression de la circulation des publications obscènes; the following year Jacques Bertillon was awarded a prize by the Académie des sciences morales et politiques for the best book on depopulation, and in 1912 the Musée sociale hosted a congress on the problems posed by neo-Malthusianism. Specialist lobbying movements also emerged to advance both the familial and populationist causes. The earliest was La Réforme sociale, founded in 1880 to popularize Le Play's ideas, and it was followed in 1894 by the creation in Montpellier of an Association de familles nombreuses and in 1908 by Captaine V.L. Maire's Ligue populaire des pères et mères de familles nombreuses.[26] But the best known of the pronatalist campaigns were those associated with the activities of Béranger, Bureau, and Bertillon, who shifted attention from the encouragement of fertility to the repression of the birth controllers.

Senator René Béranger, the most vehement opponent of the neo-Malthusians, was constantly lampooned in the birth control publications as "Père la pudeur," "le fou de la rue Pasquier," "le chef des répopulateurs." It was revealing that it was this Protestant, and not a Catholic, who led the attack on Robin and Humbert. Protestant moralists were to be in the forefront of the Third Republic's elaboration of a politically democratic, though socially conservative, ideology. In 1882 pastor Fallot founded the Ligue française de la moralité publique, which from 1893 until the First World War published under the editorship of Louis Comte a journal entitled Le relèvement sociale, which was both progressive and populationist. And it was this league, which adhered to Béranger's Fédération des sociétés contre la pornographie, that pushed for the prosecution of Humbert in Rouen in 1909.[27] Other well-known Protestants active in such matters included the economist Charles Gide, who followed Béranger as head of the Fédération, and ironically Ferdinand Buisson, the early defender of Robin, who in 1913 established the anti-Malthusian Comité démocratique d'action morale et sociale. The importance of Béranger's activities lay in the fact that from the time of Robin's first propagandizing activities the senator attempted to make such undertakings a crime. Working through his original organization, the Société centrale de protestations contre la licence des rues, he succeeded in 1898 in having the law of 2 August 1882 extended to attack not only obscenities, but also in addition any statements "contraire aux bonnes moeurs."[28] In individual cases the revised law was used against neo-Malthusians, who, for the most part, found ways of skating round it even while making their message plain. Béranger was reduced to accusing Robin of promoting promiscuity by propaganda that could not be countered given the weaknesses of the law. Harsher statutes were required.

On the Catholic side similar arguments were advanced by Paul Bureau, who led the Ligue pour le relèvement de la moralité publique, which, as the name implied, sought to counter vice in all its forms ranging from pornographic anatomical museums to birth control tracts. Bureau found his own populationist speeches often interrupted by neo-Malthusians and sought revisions in the law to silence his opponents. In addition he wanted the sale or distribution of information or appliances to facilitate abortion and contraception to be prosecuted.[29]

That revisions in the law along such lines were eventually adopted was in large part due to the activities of Jacques Bertillon, who along with A. Honnorat, Charles Richer, and E. Javal founded the Alliance nationale contre dépopulation in 1896. The Alliance, which soon changed its name to the more optimistic sounding Alliance national pour l'accroissement de la population, dropped much of the moralizing tone of the other movements and advanced social and political reasons to support the notion that neo-Malthusian propaganda had to be stamped out. The birth control campaign was presented by Bertillon as being a foreign creation imported by "criminals" to France; he specifically linked Spanish assassins to *Régénération*.[30] Within the country the subversive nature of neo-Malthusianism was proven by the fact that it was taken up by anarcho-syndicalists dedicated to the destruction of society. This linkage of sexual and political radicalism subsequently drew to the Alliance the support of wealthy businessmen. The Michelin family, for example, provided several hundred thousand francs for the publication of the *Revue de l'alliance nationale pour l'accroissement de la population française.*[31]

The brunt of the message of the *Revue* was that France needed statutes similar to the Comstock laws in the United States that would put an end to subversive sexual literature. This argument was made to factory

workers by employers before 1914 and to captive audiences of recruits by
their officers during the war. Captain Blic, an Alliance speaker whose talk
"Nous les aurons. Mais après . . . ?" was published in 1916, provided an
abbreviated account of the Alliance's doctrine. France's fertility was falling,
he asserted, because of egoism, the expense of fashion, the search for
luxury, and the erosion of the ideal of the family, undermined as it was by
alcoholism, women's work, and the sneers of intellectuals. And France's
present tragedy was caused because couples who had treasonably
weakened the country by restricting the size of their families had thus
unwittingly invited Germany to attack its neighbor. Blic's account was not
without its contradictions. On the one hand, he argued that because the
French themselves chose to practice birth control they fell victims to the
Germans; on the other he argued that those who preached
neo-Malthusianism were German agents, "les Herr Professors." To
substantiate the latter statement he noted that abortion was defended by
Sarwy, Hubl, Jauregg, and Klotz. That such activities were abetted by the
syndicalists could only confirm Blic's belief in the revolutionary origins of
birth control.

> Shout: "Halt!" to the agents of revolutions and strikes, to the sowers of
> suspicions, dissensions, and hatreds, and to the lovely preachers of free
> love and sterility; in short, to all those consciously or unconsciously
> responsible for national weakness.[32]

Population growth could be possible only if the defense of abortion and
contraception were made illegal but positive steps also had to be taken.
Blic called for changes in the tax laws, plural votes for fathers of families, a
decentralization of the economy, and an improvement of workers'
housing. Regarding the last reform, it is of interest to note that he
employed the English word "home" to designate a comfortable abode in
which a healthy and happy family could flourish.[33]

How successful were the various leagues in getting their populationist
sentiments translated into legislation? The short answer is that though they
succeeded in focusing the public's attention on the problem few practical
results were forthcoming before the First World War. Measures to support
population growth started coming before the Senate and the Chamber
from the 1880s on and found their way into the 1890 discussions of the
marriage of indigents, the 1896 proposal to simplify marriage
requirements, the 1907 debate on reducing the age of consent, the 1908
debate on the legitimation of bastards, the 1911 discussion of marriages of
minors, and the 1913 review of length of military service.[34] Much legislative
effort was put into bolstering the position of the working-class woman, the
argument being that as her condition improved, so too would the fertility

rate. The laws of 9 April 1881 and 20 July 1895 that established postal savings banks for women's small deposits, the law of 20 July 1886 providing national retirement funds as another place in which money could be removed from the control of the husband, the law of 1 April 1898 that permitted married women to join mutual aid societies without the husband's consent, and the law of 13 July 1907 giving the wife control over her own salary or income were all aimed at protecting the working woman's "dowry," that is to say, the money she herself earned. At the same time, however, the type of work she could do was restricted by the law of 2 November 1892. Moreover, she was forbidden to work at all during the last stages of pregnancy by the laws of 27 November 1909 and 17 June 1913.[35] The purpose of these laws was to protect fetal life but their critics commented that depriving women of work would make them all the more intent on limiting fertility. The acts guaranteed that a woman could return to her employment after confinement, but there was no provision of a national maternity system to make up for the wages lost by those forbidden to work.

The realization that only some form of social assistance could make any meaningful impact on the family strategies of the poor was slow in being grasped by deputies. The shock of the census reports for the years 1901–1911 helped to bring the idea home. Births fell from 857,000 in 1901 to 777,000 in 1910, from 22 per thousand to 19.5 per thousand, and this decline was viewed as all the more appalling, inasmuch as by 1911 the 776,000 deaths actually exceeded the 742,000 births.[36] It was in this context that French family legislation finally began to appear. In 1913 aid was offered to poor families with four or more children and to officers and noncommissioned officers for the third and every additional child under the age of sixteen. In 1917 these benefits were extended to all civil servants. In 1916 some employers began to provide *allocations familiales* to their workers, and the law of 29 June 1918 foresaw the state's taking similar steps to aid natality. In 1920 medals were offered to mothers of large families and reductions offered on train fares and taxes. In 1923 the aid to poor mothers now began with the arrival of the third child. For the masses, however, government assistance would not be a reality until the 1930s.[37]

The argument could be made that because the fertility rate did not respond to such positive measures the government felt forced to fall back on the negative tack of restricting access to abortion and contraception. The reality of the situation was that the campaign for new laws against birth control propaganda had begun well before the family legislation was on the books. Those who pushed for such laws held that the restriction of family size was neither involuntary nor completely volitional. In their eyes the masses had been led astray and had to be reeducated. In short, depopulation was attributed by many conservatives to some sort of conspiracy. For Couturier and Deherme the Masons were responsible, for Faguet and Vuillermet it was the Jews, for the writers noted in the opening pages of chapter ten it was the feminists, and for all the depopulationists it was the birth control propagandists.[38] To compound the guilt of the latter, they were accused by Blet, Roux, Bertillon, Leroy-Beaulieu, and Roya of combining their defense of contraception with the justification of abortion.[39]

The difficulty facing those deputies sympathetic to the populationists' argument was that while there was no law specifically dealing with contraception, there was a law on abortion of such severity that most juries refused to convict. Because of the constant changes of ministries in the decade before the war and the complicated question of how one was at the same time to increase penalties for one sort of birth control while easing those for another, the deputies found the going difficult. In 1902 Waldeck Rousseau, at the request of 133 senators acting on behalf of the Alliance national, set up an extra-parliamentary commission on depopulation. The commission met in 1902 and again in 1904. Under Émile Combes it continued intermittently to meet, and in 1905 the Prime Minister assured Piot that the government was concerned by the activities of the neo-Malthusians. Directives were sent to prefects, declared Combes, to have them refuse birth control advocates access to public buildings. The depopulation committee meanwhile sank from sight, though Paul Strauss did draw up a report on morality. In 1910 attempts were made by Gauthier de Clagny in the Chamber and O.M. Lannelogue in the Senate to reform the abortion law, but once again a change in ministry and the complications raised by the question of medical secrecy led to the failure of both initiatives. In 1912 another depopulation committee was chaired by L.L. Klotz, minister of finances, and more serious attention paid to the question of suppressing the neo-Malthusians. The outbreak of the war ended its sittings.[40]

But the war also ended the neo-Malthusian campaign. Both the *Malthusien* and *Génération Consciente* ceased to appear after August 1914. Eugène Humbert, true to his pacifist ideals, refused to enlist and fled to Spain. Gabriel Giroud attempted to carry on the fight by publishing *Le néo-malthusien* in 1916; further issues were banned by the authorities. Thus, when the conservative government returned to the question after the war, there was no organized birth control movement, the syndicalist forces had exhausted themselves, and the center-left parties which had dominated the administrations of the first decade of the century were in disarray. Meeting little opposition the populationists rammed through the law of 31 July 1920. This legislation left untouched the severe law already dealing with abortion — article 317 — but extensively widened the description of activities which could make one an accessory to the crime. As far as contraception was concerned, the law now held that jail terms of one to six months were to be meted out for the sale, distribution, or even discussion of contraceptive techniques. Clearly, the laws were aimed more at those who recommended the restriction of births than at those who followed such advice.[41]

Were the laws effective? The answer depends on what standard of measurement one employs. Neither the economic inducements of family grants nor the criminalization of neo-Malthusian propaganda had any obvious impact on the fertility rate. It continued to fall. French population growth was, with the exception of Ireland's, the slowest in Europe. Between 1900 and 1939 it increased 3 percent while in Germany it grew 36 percent, in Italy 33 percent, and in the United Kingdom 23 percent. And even the growth that France enjoyed was a result, as many had predicted, of foreign immigration. Total population increased from forty million in 1914 to forty-two million in 1939, but the number of foreigners — Italians, Belgians, and Spaniards — exceeded two million. The baby boom in the period 1920–1925 raised the birth rate back to a prewar level of 19.7 per thousand, but in 1926–1930 it fell to 18.2 per thousand, in 1931–1935 to 16.5 per thousand, and in 1936–1938 to 14.8 per thousand, leaving the country with the lowest fertility in the world.[42] As far as influencing population growth was concerned, the laws clearly had failed.

In a political sense, however, the laws were successful. The neo-Malthusian movement was crushed. For many this was sufficient. Depopulation had become for nationalists at the turn of the century a code word for the decadence of society. The tensions, anxieties, and fears of those defending the status quo were accordingly focused on the neo-Malthusians, who came to be held responsible for a vast range of problems ranging from the emergence of independent women to the declining ability of the nation to defend itself. It was for this reason that the the neo-Malthusians were attacked from so many sides. Who would not be against the depopulation and degeneration of the country? Obviously, those who sincerely believed in the necessity of large families were opposed to Robin and Humbert, but the populationist camp was mainly filled by members of the middle class who had already been successful in controlling family size. Only the poor, the unlucky, and the ignorant would need the sort of information proffered by Robin, and they were not the sort likely to influence politicians.

A close reading of the debates reveals that legislators were in fact more concerned by loss of discipline than by loss of births. The latter was taken as a symptom of the former. Combining reformist and repressive measures in the area of family law, successive French governments demonstrated by their actions that maintenance of control over women and workers ranked higher in their estimation than population growth. It is only by viewing the law of 31 July 1920 in this light that it makes any real sense. The law was an attack not on the causes of the decline of fertility but on a means of controlling fertility. A vice taken to symbolize the problems of the age was therefore legislated against, but the real causes of the social transformation that led to a drop in births were not touched. There must have been many deputies who voted for the law knowing that it could have no positive impact on population growth but content with the understanding that it would at least silence the sexual subversives. That the law had limited application is apparent from the fact that it made no mention of the main form of contraception, coitus interruptus. Nor did it outlaw sheaths, the primary mechanical contraceptives used by men. Such devices were regarded as essential for protection against venereal disease. The law was thus not only class-biased, inasmuch as it struck out at the self-appointed sex educators of the masses, but it was also sex-biased, in that only abortion and women's forms of contraception fell under its jurisdiction.

Some sympathetic to the regime have argued that the government was goaded into the passage of unnecessarily stringent laws on contraception and abortion because the anarchists and libertarians who took over the birth control movement had turned a simple demographic discussion into a political issue.[43] There is an element of truth in this argument and it raises the question of why neo-Malthusianism was so closely associated with anticlericalism, antimilitarism, and syndicalism. In answer to this question, the first chapters of this book examined the reasons for the hostility of priests, doctors, secular moralists, and socialists toward birth control. The beginnings of what one might call a respectable birth control lobby began to form within the medical profession at the turn of the century. In the previous discussions of Robin's and Humbert's movements, we noted in passing the involvement of doctors such as Lutaud, Darricarrère, Elosu, Gottschalk, Mascaux, Meslier, and Wylm. Such sympathizers still formed a tiny minority of the profession. Some such as Montalban continued to recommend the purported rhythm method; most like Castelnau, Corre, Garnier, and Marrin publicly condemned all forms of contraception.[44] What was striking, however, was the appearance of a new generation of eugenically minded technicians such as Edouard Toulouse, Henri Fischer, Sicard de Plauzoles, and Auguste Forel of Zurich, who argued that only by the provision of medically supervised birth control could one produce a healthy, efficient work force.[45] It was this sort of argument that in America and Britain would win the birth control movements the support of wealthy philanthropists interested in maintaining social order. In France medical scientists arrived too late to turn the neo-Malthusian movement to their own purposes. It began and ended as a libertarian crusade.

What happened to the birth controllers? Eugène Humbert, upon his return from Spain, was condemned in 1921 to five years in prison for evasion of military service; his wife, Jeanne Humbert, was jailed for her neo-Malthusian activities. The Humberts and Gabriel Giroud would do what they could in the interwar period to keep the world informed of the fall in French fertility, but there was little scope for activity within France. Robin did not see the final wave of repression, having committed suicide in 1912. His last act was well thought out and taken for the purpose of sparing himself unnecessary pain. Just as he believed that births should be consciously planned, so too he defended the individual's right to determine his own death. Laura and Paul Lafargue had ended their lives out of a similar belief, as would Dr. J. Rutgers, leader of the Dutch neo-Malthusian League, and Ernest Verliac, founder of the Group ouvrier néo-malthusien. Robin's suicide confirmed his enemies' conviction that the man was not only immoral but mad; it impressed his friends as a sign of his intense desire once again to put theory into practice.[46]

Notes

INTRODUCTION

1. Michel Foucault, *Histoire de la sexualité* (Paris, 1976); Jacques Donzelot, *La Police des familles* (Paris, 1977).
2. The following works were brought to my attention at too late a date for their interpretations to be included in the present study: James R. Lehning, *The Peasants of Marlhes: Economic Development and Family Organization in Nineteenth Century France* (Chapel Hill, 1980); Francis Ronsin, *La Grève des ventres: propagande néo-malthusienne et baisse de la natalité en France, 19e-20e siècles* (Paris, 1980); Charles Sowerine, *Les Femmes et la socialisme* (Paris, 1978); Robert Wheaton and T.K. Hareven, eds., *Family and Sexuality in French History* (Philadelphia, 1980).

CHAPTER ONE

1. See Joseph J. Spengler, *France Faces Depopulation* (Duke University Press, 1938).
2. Léonce de Lavergne, *Revue des deux mondes* (1 April 1857), p. 489.
3. Paul E. Vincent, "French Demography in the Eighteenth Century," *Population Studies* (1947–1948), 44.
4. J. Overbeek, *History of Population Theories* (Rotterdam, 1974).
5. A. Quetelet, *Sur l'homme et le développement de ses facultés, ou essai de physique sociale* (Paris, 1835). See also Sir Francis d'Ivernois, *Sur la fécondité et la mortalité proportionelles des peuples* (Geneva, 1836); M.A. Legoyt, *Journal des économistes* 13 (1857), 321-336; Joseph Garnier, *Journal des économistes* 14 (1857), 340-351.
6. See C.M. Raudot, *De la décadence de la France* (Paris, 1850); Léonce de Lavergne, *Revue des deux mondes* (1 July 1855, 1 April 1857); M. Prévost-Paradol, *La nouvelle France* (Paris, 1868), pp. 413–415.
7. Frédéric Le Play, *Les ouvriers européens* . . . (Paris, 1855).
8. For what follows see J.L. Flandrin, *Familles, parenté, maison, sexualité, dans l'ancienne société* (Paris, 1976), Marcel Lachiver, *La Population de Meulan du XVIIIe siècle* (Paris, 1969); J. Hajnal, "European Marriage Patterns in Perspective," in *Population in History*, D.V. Glass and D.E.C. Eversley, eds., (London, 1965), pp. 101–143.
9. Gérard Bouchard, *Le Village immobile: Sennely-en-Sologne au XVIIIe siècle* (Paris, 1972).
10. A. Zink, *Azereix, la vie d'une communauté rurale à la fin du 18e siècle* (Paris, 1969), p. 73; Jean Meyer, "La limitation des naissances en France à l'époque moderne," in *Histoire sociale* 10 (1977), 259-260.
11. Louis Henry, "Fécondité des mariages dans le quart sud-ouest de la France de 1720 à 1829," *Annales E.S.C.* 4–6 (1972), 1001–1003.
12. Flandrin stresses the importance of taboos during nursing; Lawrence Stone asserts that no such taboos existed in England. Stone, *The Family, Sex and Marriage in England 1500–1800* (London, 1977), p. 64. It should be noted that restriction of family size

was also an effect of both a low level of fecundity due to maternal malnutrition and fetal loss through stillbirths; both factors are obviously difficult to determine with any precision.

13. See Louis Henry, "The Population of France in the 18th Century," and Pierre Goubert, "French Population Between 1500 and 1700," in Glass and Eversley, eds., *Population*, pp. 457–473; Roland Mousnier, "Études sur la population de la France au XVIIe siècle," *XVIIe Siècle* (1952), pp. 527–542; Pierre Goubert, *Beauvais et le Beauvaisis de 1600 à 1730* (Paris, 1960); Olwen Hufton, *The Poor of Eighteenth Century France* (Oxford, 1974).

14. J. Bourgeois-Pichat, "The General Development of the Population of France since the Eighteenth Century," in Glass and Everseley, eds., *Population*, pp. 473–506.

15. E. van de Walle, "Alone in Europe: The French Fertility Decline until 1850," Charles Tilly, ed., *Historical Studies of Changing Fertility* (Princeton, 1978), pp. 257–288.

16. Louis Henry, *Anciennes familles génévoises* (Paris, 1956); L. Henry and C. Levy, "Ducs et pairs sous l'ancienne régime, caractéristique démographique d'une caste," *Population*, (1960), pp. 807–830; R. Gresset, *Le Monde judiciare à Besançon de la conquête à la révolution française, 1674–1789* (Lille, 1975); Thomas F. Sheppard, *Lourmarin in the Eighteenth Century: A Study of a French Village* (Baltimore, 1971) p. 38; Marcel Lachiver, "Fécondité légitime et contraception dans la région parisienne," in Société de démographie historique, *Sur la population française au XVIIIe siècle et au XIXe siècle* (Paris, 1973), pp. 383–401.

17. See, for example, Flandrin, *Familles*; Stone, *The Family*, and Edward Shorter, *The Making of the Modern Family* (London, 1976).

18. Sheppard, *Lourmarin*, pp. 46–47.

19. See J. Houdaille, "La Fécondité des mariages de 1670 à 1829 dans le quart nord-est de la France," *Annales de démographie historique*, (1976), pp. 360–361.

20. P. Ariès, *Centuries of Childhood: A Social History of Family Life* (New York, 1962), p. 413.

21. Flandrin, *Familles*, pp.220–221.

22. Flandrin, *Familles*, pp. 214–217. Jean Sauvy, *A General Theory of Population* (New York, 1969), p. 362.

23. On the decline of social constraints on lower class sexual and marital behavior see Cissie Fairchilds, "Masters and Servants in Eighteenth Century Toulouse," *Journal of Social History* (1978), pp. 368–393 and "Female Sexual Attitudes and the Rise of Illegitimacy: A Case Study," *Journal of Interdisciplinary History* 4 (1978), pp. 627–667.

24. Edward Shorter, "Female Emancipation, Birth Control, and Fertility in European History," *American Historical Review* 78 (1973), 605–640; Etienne van de Walle and Samuel H. Preston, "Mortalité de l'enfance au XIXe siècle à Paris et dans le départment de la Seine," *Population* 29 (1974), 89 ff.; J. Dupaquier and M. Lachiver, "Sur les débuts de la contraception en France ou les deux malthusianismes," *Annales E.S.C.* 24,6 (1969), 1398–1399; George D. Sussman, "The Wet-nursing Business in Nineteenth Century France," *French Historical Studies* 9 (1975), 304—328.

25. Patricia James, *Population Malthus: His Life and Times* (London, 1979), p. 387.

26. See also James Reed, *From Private Vice to Public Virtue: The Birth Control Movement and American Society Since 1830* (New York, 1978), p. 387.

27. Dr. Auguste Lutaud, *Les Néo-Malthusiens* (1891), p. 2.

28. P.J. Boudier de Villermet, *L'Ami des femmes* (1758), p. 139; see also L. Populus, *Dissertation sur l'allaitement* (Paris, 1815), p. 22.

29. Charles Loudon, *Solution du problème de la population et la subsistence* (Paris, 1842); Marc Leproux, *Du berceau à la tombe* (Paris, 1959), p. 10 and see also M. Rouxel, *Journal des économistes* (March 1886), pp. 419–429.

30. Laurent Joubert, *Erreurs populaires au fait de la médecine et regime de santé* (Paris, 1776), pp. 167–168.

31. Dr. Venel, *Essai sur la santé et sur l'éducation médicinale des filles destinées au mariage* (Paris, 1776), pp. 65–66.

32. Nicolas Venette, *La Génération de l'homme ou tableau de l'amour conjugal* (Amsterdam, 1778) 1:305. See also condemnations of forbidden positions in *Père Féline, Catéchisme des gens mariés* (Paris, 1782), p. 7. Dr. J.F. Giraud, *Confidence à une jeune épouse* (Marseilles, 1834), pp. 31–33.

33. Dr. Dartigues, *De l'amour expérimentale ou des causes d'adultère chez la femme au XIXe siècle* (Paris, 1887), pp. 136–137.

34. Dr. Forel, *La Question sexuelle exposée aux adultes cultivées* (Paris, 1911), p. 486.

35. Henri Thulié, *La Femme* (Paris, 1885), p. 319.

36. Jacques Bertillon, *La Dépopulation de la France* (Paris, 1911).

37. On Place see Angus McLaren, *Birth Control in Nineteenth Century England* (London, 1978), p. 55. See also Dr. Mayer, *Des Rapports conjugaux* (Paris, 1857), p. 144.

38. Joseph Garnier, *Journal des économistes* (1863), p. 148–155; Emile Zola, *Earth* (New York, 1962), p. 98; Dartigues, *De l'amour*, p.123.; Lutaud, *Le Néo-Malthusiens;* Boismoreau, *Coutumes médicales et superstitions populaires du bocage vendéen* (Paris, 1911), pp. 45–46.

39. Dr. Raymond Belbèze, *La Neurasthénie rurale* (Paris, 1911), p. 115. Belbèze wrote "coïtus reservatus" when he must have meant "coïtus interruptus." The former practice was employed by members of the Oneida colony in the state of New York but there are very few references to it in France.

40. J. Stengers, "Les Pratiques anticonceptionelles dans le mariage au XIXe et au XXe siècle: Problèmes humaines et attitudes religieuses," *Revue belge de philosophie et d'histoire* 49 (1971), 480. In the twentieth century this maneuver was referred to as "fireworks on the lawn" and "jumping off the train while it is still running." See Sanche de Gramont, *The French: Portrait of a People* (New York, 1969), p. 406.

41. M.B. Lavigne, *Histoire du Blagnac* (Toulouse, 1875), pp. 372–373.

42. Flandrin, *Familles*, p. 209.

43. See Hans Ferdy, "Contribution à l'étude historique du 'Coecal Condom'," *Gazette médicale* 12 (1905), 535–537.

44. Jean Astruc, *A Treatise of the Venereal Disease* (London, 1737), 1:299.

45. Philippe Ricord, *Traité practique des maladies vénériennes* (Paris, 1858), p. 544.

46. Cited by G.J. Witkowski, *La Génération humaine* (Paris, 1881), p. 169.

47. Charles Londe, *Nouveaux Éléments d'hygiène* (Paris, 1827) 2:412–413.

48. *Dictionnaire des sciences médicales* vol. XLVII (Paris, 1820), p. 329.

49. Mm. Bertherand and Duchesne, "Des Boyaux dits preservatifs," *Annales de la société de médecine de Lyon* 25 (1877), 201–217.

50. Lutaud, *Les Néo-Malthusiens*, p. 5; Forel, *Question*, p. 487; Brennus, *Amour et Sécurité* (Paris, 1906), Dartigues, *L'Amour*, p. 136.

51. Mathurin Regnier, *Les Satyrs* (1609) in *Oeuvres complètes* (Paris, 1958), pp. 160–161.

52. Henri Estienne, *L'Introduction au traité de la conformité des merveilles anciennes avec les modernes* (Paris, 1566), p. 256.

53. Richard Carlile, *Every Woman's Book* (London, 1826).

54. Lutaud, *Les Néo-Malthusiens*, p. 6.
55. Drs. Bardet and Dufau, "L'Exercice de la pharmacie dans ses rapports avec la réproduction," *Bulletin général de thérapeutique* 160 (1910), 12.
56. Arthur Young, *Travels in France and Italy During the Years 1787, 1788, and 1789* (London, n.d.), p. 324.
57. Marc Colombat de l'Isère, *A Treatise on the Disease and Special Hygiene of Females*, trans. Charles Meigs (Philadelphia, 1945), p 556. See also Lutaud, *Les Néo-Malthusiens*, p. 5; Brennus, *Armour*, p. 64. Forel, *Question*, p. 485.
58. Robert Michels, *Sexual Ethics: A Study of Borderland Questions* (London, 1914), p. 262.
59. See Bertier de Sauvigny, "Population Movements and Political Change in Nineteenth Century France," *Review of Politics* 19 (1957), 37–47; Marcel Reinhard, et al., *Histoire général de la population mondiale* (Paris, 1968); Charles Pouthas, *La Population française pendant la première moitié du XIXᵉ siècle* (Paris, 1956); Colin Dyer, *Population and Society in Twentieth Century France* (London, 1978), pp. 22–28.
60. Joseph J. Spengler, "Notes on France's Response to Her Declining Rate of Demographic Growth," in Spengler, ed., *Demographic Analysis* (New York, 1956).
61. Etienne van de Walle, *The Female Population of France in the Nineteenth Century: A Reconstitution of Eighty-two Departments* (Princeton, 1974), chap. 7.
62. In fact, by the end of the nineteenth century in an area such as Bordeaux the completed family size of lower-class families was, because of their relatively high death rates, only slightly larger than those of the middle class. Employees had the lowest birth rates and industrial workers the highest. See Pierre Guillaume, *La Population de Bordeaux au XIXᵉ siècle essai d'histoire sociale* (Paris, 1972), pp. 201–203 ff.

CHAPTER TWO

1. For overviews of the issue see Philippe Ariès, *Histoire de populations françaises et de leurs attitudes devant la vie depuis le 18ᵉ siècle* (Paris, 1971), pp. 312–321; Joseph J. Spengler, *France Faces Depopulation* (Durham, North Carolina, 1938), pp. 173–174; J.L. Flandrin, *L'Église et le contrôle des naissances* (Paris, 1970); John T. Noonan, *Contraception: A History of its Treatment by Catholic Theologians and Canonists* (Cambridge, Mass., 1965); Theodore Zeldin, "The Conflict of Moralities. Confession, Sin and Pleasure in the Nineteenth Century," Zeldin, ed., *Conflicts in French Society* (London, 1970), pp. 13–51.
2. A. Perrenoud, "Malthusianisme et protestantisme," *Annales E.S.C.* 29 (1974), 975–988.
3. M. Mesnard, *Catéchisme du diocèse de Nantes* (Nantes, 3rd ed. 1689) p.345, cited by Jean Meyer, "Limitation des naissances en France à l'époque moderne," *Histoire sociale/Social History* 10 (1977), 251.
4. Père Féline, *Catéchisme des gens mariés* (Caen, 1782), pp. 41–42.
5. Abbé Pierre Jaubert, *Des Causes de la dépopulation et des moyens d'y remédier* (Londres, 1767), pp. vi, 39.
6. On the eighteenth-century church see Jean Queniart, *Les Hommes, l'église, et Dieu dans la France du 18ᵉ siècle* (Paris, 1978), pp. 233–288.
7. J.P. Duroselle, *Les Débuts du catholicisme sociale en France, 1822–1870* (Paris, 1951), pp. 40, 65.

8. Féline, *Catéchisme*, pp. 7–8; and see also Julia Dominique, "Sur les moeurs périgourdines," *Annales de démographie historique*, (1971), pp. 417–420.

9. On one aspect of the church's difficulties see François Isambert, "L'Attitude religieuse des ouvriers français au milieu du 19ᵉ siècle," *Archives de sociologie des religions* 6 (1958), 7–35.

10. On the argument that the laxity of eighteenth-century confessors following Ligouri's line aided in the spread of birth control, see André Armengaud, *La Famille et l'enfant en France et Angleterre du 16ᵉ au 18ᵉ siècles: aspect démographiques* (Paris, 1975). For the more ironical thesis that contraception was in fact furthered by the rigorism of Jansenist teachings, which in denigrating the sexual act provided an unanticipated apology for those who chose to view the practice of coitus interruptus as a form of asceticism, see Pierre Chaunu, "Réflexions sur la démographie normande," *Mélanges publiés en l'honneur de Marcel Reinhard* (Paris, 1973), pp. 97–118; Flandrin, *Familles*, pp. 226–229.

11. Hélène Bergues, ed., *La Prévention des naissances dans la famille* (Paris, 1960), p. 229.

12. See also the discussion of "L'onanisme conjugal" in the work of the doctor-priest P.J.C. Debreyne, *Essai sur la théologie morale* (Paris, 1842), pp. 174–187. Debreyne's main concern was to prevent women with small families from being driven from the church and he accordingly justified confessors in downplaying the woman's involvement in coitus interruptus by declaring the husband the main culprit and the wife a mere accessory; he crudely likened her to the accomplice of a thief who holds the loot.

13. Noonan, *Contraception*, pp. 398–399.

14. Dr. Jean-Ennemond Dufieux, *Nature et virginité* (Paris, 1854), p. 243.

15. Dufieux, *Nature,*, p. 454.

16. Augustine, *The Moral of the Manichees* cited by Noonan, *Contraception*, p. 120.

17. Un libre penseur (author's *nom de plume*), *L'Amour; Renversement des propositions de M. Michelet* (Paris, 1859), p. 194.

18. Noonan, *Contraception*, pp. 438–439.

19. Gustave Le Bon, *Physiologie de la génération de l'homme* (Paris, 1868), pp. 180–201. Le Bon states that Gousset's response came in a letter — not to Dr. Avard as asserts Noonan — but to a Dr. Varardet.

20. See the review of Lecomte in *Nouvelle revue théologique* 5 (1873) 522–532.

21. The author of a recent history of Belgian fertility seems to believe that Lecomte was discussing an effective form of contraception. See R.J. Lesthaegue, *The Decline of Belgian Fertility, 1800–1970* (Princeton, 1977), pp. 135–136.

22. H.A. Frégier, *Des Classes dangereuses de la population dans les grandes villes* (Paris, 1840), 1:326–335.

23. Abbé Corbière, "Le Malthusianisme," *L'Ami de la religion* (27 May 1858), p. 479; (29 May 1858), p. 499. The militant Catholic journalist Louis Veuillot presented Catholicism in the 1860s as the only effective force against depopulation. See Georges Deherme, *Croître ou disparaître* (Paris, 1910), p. 62 and L. Mounier, "Le Principle de population: réfutation du malthusianisme," *Revue catholique des institutions et du droit* 3 (1873–1874), 162–176, 299–230. An early attack on Malthusians in *Instruction pastorale sur les rapports de la charité avec la foi* (1843) by Archbishop D.A. Affre of Paris, is cited in Dufieux, *Nature*, p. 455.

24. See, for example, Père Charles Daniel, *Le Mariage chrètien* (Paris, 1870), Eugène Buisson, *L'homme, la famille, et la société considérés dans leurs rapports avec le progrès moral de l'humanité* (Paris, 1857), 2:135–140; A. Egron, *De l'influence du christianisme sur l'esprit de famille* (Paris, 1844), pp. 18–55; Abbé Martinet, *La Science sociale au point de vue des faits* (Paris, 1851), p. 398.

25. L.E. Bautain, *Philosophie morale* (Paris, 1842), 1:234. Bautain concluded on page 382: "The most faithful marriages are generally the most fruitful."

26. Marie-Jean Guyau, *L'Irreligion de l'avenir* (Paris, 1887), p. 282.

27. Guyau, *L'Irreligion*, p. 283.

28. On the eighteenth-century critiques of clerical celibacy, see Flandrin, *L'Église*, p.80; for the nineteenth century, see Henri Guillemin, *Le Jocelyn de Lamartine* (Paris, 1936), pp.491–502; for P.L. Courier, see his *Oeuvres complètes* (Paris, 1836), 2: pp. 52ff. Anticlericals later in the nineteenth century adopted the tack of simply republishing the passages from confessors' manuals dealing with sensitive sexual issues to prove the charge of church interference in marriage. Sections of the *Compendium theologiae moralis* and *Casus conscientiae* were contained for example in Paul Bert, *La Morale des Jésuits* (Paris, 1880).

29. Joseph de Maistre, *Du pape* (Paris, 1821), 2:110.

30. Dufieux, *Nature*, pp. 468–470. Dr. Paul Diday, *Du célibat religieux* (Paris, 1861).

31. For attacks on celibacy see Arsène Dumont, *Dépopulation et civilization* (Paris, 1890); Debury (G. Rossignol), *Un Pays de célibataires et de fils unique* (Paris, 1913); Jean Boillot, *La Pays de la revanche et le pays des milliards: Réponse au Dr. Rommel* (Paris, 1886); for defenses see Camille Ract, *Natalité* (Paris, 1901), D.M. Couturier, *Demain, la dépopulation de la France, craintes et espérances* (Paris, 1901).

32. Cited by Noonan, *Contraception*, p. 414.

33. Cited by A. Armengaud, *Les Français et Malthus* (Paris, 1975), p. 130.

34. Etienne Lamy, "La flamme qui ne doit pas s'éteindre," *Revue des deux mondes* 42 (1917), 852.

35. Alfred Krug, *Pour la repopulation et contre la vie chère* (Paris, 1918), p. 33.

36. Cited by Noonan, *Contraception*, p. 422.

37. The Bishop followed up on his observation with the warning, "Take care! the detestable sin which empties homes compromises at the same time the nation's security." Monseigneur Gibier, *Patrie* (Paris, 1919), p. 172. For an earlier example of much the same sentiments see Le T.R.P. J-M-L Monsabré, *Le Mariage* (Paris, 1887), pp. 166–175 and Y.M. Hilaire, "Les Missions intérieures face à la déchristianisation pendant la seconde moitié du 19ᵉ siècle dans la région du Nord," *Revue du Nord* 46 (1964), 59.

CHAPTER THREE

1. François Foy, *Manuel d'hygiène* (Paris, 1845), pp. 571–72; and see also J.B.T. Serrurier, *Du mariage considéré dans ses rapports physiques et moraux* (Paris, 1845). For a contrasting view which held that family illness had to be seen as messages from God see Mme. de Gasparin, *Le Mariage au point de vue chrétienne* (Paris, 1843), 3:149.

2. Jean Cruveilhier, *Des Devoirs et de la moralité du médecin* (Paris, 1837), pp. 23–24.

3. It was noted by Dr. Aulagnier that both doctors and charlatans focused their attention on women and children whose chronic ailments, unlike the precipitous diseases of the male, required continual attention. Dr. Aulagnier, *Nouveau recueil d'observations et de consultations sur les maladies des femmes* (Paris, 1821), p. iv. See also P.S. Thouvenel, *Essai sur les devoirs publics et particuliers du médecin* (Paris, 1806), p. 32.

4. B.J.B. Buchez and U. Trélat, *Précis élémentaire d'hygiène* (Paris, 1825) p. 24; see also H. Crosilhes, *Hygiène et maladies des femmes* (Paris, 1850), p. 2.

5. Dr. Desbruères, *Hygiène des femmes* (Paris, 1845), pp. xiv, xvi.

6. Jules Michelet, *L'Amour* (Paris, 1889 [1st edition, 1858]), p. 52.

7. Desbruères, *Hygiène*, pp. xv, xvii; and see also Dr. M.H. Chomet, *Conseils aux femmes sur leur santé* (Paris, 1846), p. 5.

8. Thouvenel, *Essai*, p. 32.

9. Louis Huart, *Physiologie du médecin* (Paris, 1840), p. 78.

10. Jules Michelet, *Du prêtre, de la femme, de la famille* (Paris, 1854), p. 245; on the danger of the priest see also Mme. de Casamajor [Emile Barrault], *Pathologie du mariage* (Paris, 1847), pp. 117–120.

11. Philippe Hecquet, *L'Indécence aux hommes d'accoucher les femmes* (Trevoux, 1708), pp. 85–86. See also Dehaut, *Les Médecins dévoilés* (Paris, 1846), p. 21 for an attack on doctors' attempts to replace midwives. On the general danger of the doctor/female patient relationship, see P. Belouino, *La Femme: physiologie, histoire, morale* (Paris, 1860), p. 35, and the novel of Edouard Alletz, *Maladies du siècle* (Paris, 1835).

12. J.J. Rousseau, *Emile ou l'éducation* in *Oeuvres complètes* (Paris, 1971), 3:25.

13. Honoré de Balzac, *Physiologie du mariage* (Paris, 1835), p. 338.

14. Huart, *Physiologie*, p. 78.

15. Michelet, *L'Amour*, p. 163.

16. Ibid., p. 222.

17. Jules Michelet, *La Femme* (Paris, 1860), pp. 420–423.

18. Étienne Cabet, *Voyage en Icarie* (Paris, 1842), p. 115.

19. Dr. Ratier, "Onanisme," *Encyclopédie des gens du monde* (Paris, 1844), 18:693.

20. Philippe Ricord, *Traité practique des maladies vénériennes* (Paris, 1858, [1st edition, 1838]), p. 541.

21. Colombat de l'Isère, *A Treatise on the Diseases and Special Hygiene of Females*, trans., Ch. Meigs (Philadelphia, 1845), p. 544. See also Belouino, *La Femme*, p. 424; M. Bureaud-Riofrey, *Education physique des jeunes filles* (Paris, 1835); Dr. D'Huc, *Hygiène des femmes* (Paris, 1841), p. 32.

22. J.J. Virey, *De la femme* (Paris, 1823), p. 96.

23. Louis Seraine, *De la santé des gens mariés* (Paris, 1865), p. 26.

24. C. Lachaise, *Hygiène physiologique de la femme* (Paris, 1825), pp. 30, 118, and see also Dr. P. Roussel, *Système physique et moral de la femme* (Paris, 1805), p. 119.

25. Lachaise, *Hygiène*, p. 121; cf. M*** (author's *nom de plume*), *Hygiène des dames* (Paris, 1819), p. 30.

26. Colombat de l'Isère, *A Treatise*, pp. 544–45. Dr. Audin-Rouvière stated that leeches were even used to hasten menstruation in his *L'Oracle de la santé ou l'art de se bien porter* (Paris, 1829), p. 45.

27. Jean Houdaille, *Essai physiologique sur la femme* (Paris, 1820), p. 11. For older views of menstruation see also Nicolas Venette, *La Génération de l'homme ou tableau de l'amour conjugal* (Amsterdam, 1778), 2:84ff.

28. F.A. Pouchet, *Théorie positive de l'ovulation spontanée et de la fécondation* (Paris, 1847), pp. 275–277.

29. Crosilhes, *Hygiène*, pp. 5–6.

30. Michelet, *L'Amour*, pp. 183, 185.

31. Henri Guillemin, *Hugo et la sexualité* (Paris, 1954), p. 13.

32. Virey, *La Femme*, p. 98; cf. D'Huc. *Hygiène*, p. 58.

33. Lachaise, *Hygiène physiologique*, p. 223; Charles Londe, *Nouveaux élémens d'hygiène* (Paris, 1827), 1:111–12.

34. Virey, *La Femme*, pp. 94, 182ff; see also H. Crosilhes, *Le Médecin de familles* (Paris, 1849), p. 688.

35. Dargir, *L'Hymen, réformateur des abus du mariage ou le code conjugal dans l'univers* (Paris, 1756), p. 6.

36. Desbruères, *Hygiène des femmes*, p. 16; L.F.E. Bergeret, *Des Fraudes dans l'accomplissement des fonctions génératrices* (Paris, 1868); Gustave Le Bon, *Physiologie de la génération de l'homme* (Paris, 1868), p. 154.

37. Buchez and Trélat, *Précis*, p. 220; see also L. Rostan, *Cours élémentaires d'hygiène* (Paris, 1822), 1:75.

38. Lachaise, *Hygiène physiologique*, pp. 240–241; and see also Dr. Léopold Deslandes, *De l'onanisme et des autres abus vénériens* (Paris, 1835), p. 50.

39. G.J. Barker-Benfield, "The Spermatic Economy: A Nineteenth Century View of Sexuality," *Feminist Studies*, vol. 1, no. 1. (1972): p. 53ff.

40. J.J. Virey, *Hygiène philosophique* (Paris, 1828), 1:58; see also Dr. Audin-Rouvière, *L'Oracle de la santé*, (Paris, 1829) p. 25; Dr. A. Reinvillier, *Hygiène pratique des femmes* (Paris, 1854), p. 63.

41. Venette, *La Génération de l'homme ou tableau de l'amour conjugal,* 1:170.

42. Dargir, *Hymen*, p. 26.

43. Virey, *La femme*, p. 100; and see also Rostan, *Cours*, 2:323; Buchez and Trélat, *Précis,* p. 225; M. Valentin, *Nouveau Manuel de santé ou hygiène domestique* (Paris, 1836), pp. 156–61.

44. V. Parisot, *Traité élémentaire de morale ou théorie du devoir et des devoirs* (Paris, 1842), p. 130; F. Voisin, *Des Causes morales et physiques des maladies mentales* (Paris, 1826), pp. 110–113.

45. J.H. Réveillé-Parisé, *Physiologie et hygiéne des hommes livrés au travaux de l'esprit* (Paris, 1839), 2:296; see also J.B.F. Descuret, *La Médecine des passions* (Paris, 1841), p. 484; Michel Lévy, *Traité d'hygiène publique et privée* (Paris, 1862), 1:176ff. C.F. Lallemand, *Des Pertes seminales involuntaires* (Paris, 1835–1842), 3:476.

46. Genesis, XXXVIII: 7–10.

47. The European-wide reputation of Tissot (1728–1797) as an enlightened practitioner of progressive views had been established by his publication in 1754 of *L'Innoculation justifée*. Notables who were to solicit his advice included J.J. Rousseau, Voltaire, and the young Napoleon Bonaparte. In addition to its inclusion in Tissot's collected works published in 1769, 1809–1813, and 1840, *L'Onanisme* was to appear in thirty-nine separate editions between 1760 and 1905. See Charles Eynard, *Essai sur la vie de Tissot* (Paris, 1839).

48. Auguste Tissot, *L'Onanisme* (Lausanne, 1760), pp. 3ff.

49. *L'Encyclopédie, ou dictionnaire raisonné* (Neufchatel, 1765), 10:51.

50. Ibid., p. 52.

51. Cited by Michel Foucault, *Madness and Civilization: A History of Insanity in the Age of Reason*, trans. R. Howard (New York, 1965), p. 128.

52. See E.H. Hare, "Masturbatory Insanity: The History of an Idea," *The Journal of Mental Science* (1962) 108:1–25 and René A. Spitz, "Authority and Masturbation," *The Psychoanalytical Quarterly* (1952) 21:490–527.

53. Gymnastic exercises were also lauded as a means of preventing the "dreadful vice, which tends every day to the deterioration of the human race." Peter Henry Clias, *An Elementary Course of Gymnastic Exercises* (London, 1823), p. vii. See also J.H. Réveillé-Parisé, *Gazette médical* (7 February 1835); John Duffy, "Masturbation and Clitoridectomy: A Nineteenth Century View," *Journal of the American Medical Association* (1963), 186:246–248.

54. J.B. Téraube, *Traité de la chiromanie* (Paris, 1826), pp. 165–166. The introduction of mechanical devices into the sexual realm was not restricted to the antionanists. Téraube mentions the use by miscreants of "certain instruments invented by corruption."

55. Deslandes, *De l'onanisme* (Paris, 1835), pp. 535–537.

56. Curtis, *De la virilité* (Paris, 1847), p. 122. This book first appeared in London in 1840 entitled *Manhood*.

57. R. Parry, *L'Ami discret* (Paris, 1854), pp. 83, 87. This work was first published in London as *The Secret Friend*. For a similar type of publication that circulated in France see also R.J. Brodie and Co., *The Secret Companion, A Medical Work on Onanism* (London, 1845). For English quacks who cited Tissot and the French medical profession in brochures advertising their wares see J. Hodson, *Nature's Assistant to the Restoration of Health* (London, 1795); *Dr. Ricord's Essence of Life* (London, 1860); *Dr. Paris' Treatise on Nervous Debility With New Mode of Treatment* (London, 1861).

58. Lallemand, *Des Pertes séminales involuntaires* (Paris, 1838–1842) 3:501.

59. Ibid., 1:604.

60. Ibid., 1:316.

61. See also Adouin et al, *Encyclopédie portative* (Paris, 1840), pp. 31–33. J.B.F. Descuret, *La Médecine des passions* (Paris, 1841); Dr. Meirieu and Dr., Léon Simon, *Traité élémentaire d'hygiène privée* (Paris, 1842); Dr. François Foy, *Manuel d'hygiène* (Paris, 1845); Dr. Jules Masse, *Lettres sur les maladies viriles* (Paris, 1857); Dr. Louis Seraine, *De la santé des gens mariés* (Paris, 1865).

62. Rousseau, *Émile* (Paris, 1959), 4:256. See also P.J. Boudier de Villermet, *L'Ami des femmes* (Paris, 1758), p. 139.

63. Rousseau, *Émile*, 5:698. Moheau likewise attributed the spread of contraception to women. "Rich women . . . are not the only ones who regard the propagation of the species as an old-fashioned foolishness . . . , already the deadly secrets unknown to every other animal except man have penetrated the countryside: even in the villages nature is deceived." *Recherches et considérations sur la population de la France* (Paris, 1778) 2:102.

64. J.A. Millot and A.J. Coffin-Rosny, *Le Nestor français ou guide moral et physiologique, pour conduire la jeunesse au bonheur* (Paris, 1807) 3:3–4.

65. On the importance of "vital fluids" see also Virey, *De la femme*, p. 44 and Joseph Moreau, *Les Facultés morales considérées sous la point de vue médical* (Paris, 1836), p. 148.

66. Millot and Coffin-Rosny, *Le Nestor français*, 1:290.

67. Millot and Coffin-Rosny, *Le Nestor français*, 3:385.

68. Bergeret, *Des Fraudes*, p. 161.

69. Raciborski, *De la puberté*, (Paris, 1844) intr. See also P. Cazeaux, *Traité théorique et pratique de l'art des accouchements*, 2nd ed. (Paris, 1845) and C. Négrier, *Recherches anatomiques et physiologiques sur les ovaires* (Paris, 1840).

70. Pouchet, *Théorie positif de l'ovulation spontanée*, p. 275.

71. Raciborski, *De la puberté*, p. xii.

72. Debay, *Histoire*, p. 422. Debay's *Histoire des métamorphoses humaines* went through thirteen editions, his *Philosophie du mariage* (Paris, 1849) six editions, and his *Hygiène du mariage* (Paris, 1848) forty-eight editions. The rhythm method was also publicized by Dr. Alex. Mayer, *Des Rapports conjugaux* (Paris, 1849), Dr. Francis Devay, *Hygiène des familles* (Paris, 1846), Michel Lévy, *Traité d'hygiène publique et privée* (Paris, 1844), and Dr. Charles Montalban, *La Petite Bible des jeunes epoux* (Paris, 1885).

73. Mayer, *Rapports conjugaux*, p. 142.

74. Ibid., p. 144; see also Thulié, La Femme, pp. 319–320; and L.E. Bautain, Philosophie morale (Paris, 1842) 1:234.

75. Devay, Hygiène des familles, 2:77—78.

76. Cited by Le Bon, Physiologie, p. 180; and see also Montalban, La Petite Bible, p. 102; and Raciborski's critique of Charles Loudon who believed that extended nursing was a natural means of birth control: Raciborski, De la puberté, pp. 119–21.

77. Dartigues, De l'amour,m pp. 123–24.

78. Mayer, Rapports conjugaux, p. 161.

79. "Happily the married woman cannot make herself unfruitful by her own will, she needs the husband as an accomplice: it is the latter who has all the responsibility." J.M. Guyau, L'Irréligion de l'avenir (Paris, 1887), p. 283.

80. It might be noted that the Catholic doctor Devaye, who in 1846 had publicized the rhythm method refused to discuss it in 1858 and instead fell back on the traditional solution of abstinence. Francis Devaye, Traité spécial d'hygiène des familles (Paris, 1858), p. 179. See also Dr. Jean-Ennemond Dufieux, Nature et Virginité: Considérations physiologiques sur le célibat religieux (Paris, 1854), p. 407.

81. In 1840 the Journal des femmes began a column written by a doctor on women's illnesses; such a column was to become a regular feature of almost every publication aimed at a female audience. See Evelyn Sullerot, Histoire de la press féminine en France des origines à 1848 (Paris, 1966), p. 182. By the latter half of the century feminists were attacking the medical arguments of female inferiority. See, for example, André Léo, La Femme et les moeurs (Poissy, 1869), p. 50 and Adèle Esquiros, L'Amour (Paris, 1860), p. 84. In a later chapter the response of women to the medical profession's portrayal of their "sickly" state will be examined. For a study of the American case along somewhat similar lines, see Ann Douglas Wood, " 'The Fashionable Disease': Women's Complaints and Their Treatment in Nineteenth Century America," Journal of Interdisciplinary History (1973) 4:25–52.

CHAPTER FOUR

1. Friedrich Grimm, Correspondance littéraire, philosophique et critique (Paris, 1813) 1:390–391; cf. 5:318–319.

2. Ange Goudar, Les Interêts de la France mal entendus (Amsterdam, 1756), 1:263, 268.

3. S.N.H. Linguet, Théorie des loix civiles, ou principes fondamentaux de la société (Londres, 1767) 1:222–223.

4. L.G. Dubuat-Nançay, Éléments de la politique (Londres, 1773), 1:146.

5. M. Messance, Nouvelles recherches sur la population de la France (Paris, 1788), p. 27.

6. "A great deal of eighteenth-century thought would assume a different complexion, if it was constantly remembered that though a philosophy of protest, revolt and spontaneity, eighteenth-century philosophy as already hinted, was intensely aware of the challenge to redefine the guarantees of social cohesion and morality. The philosophes were most anxious to show that not they, but their opponents were the anarchists from the point of view of the natural order." J.L. Talmon, The Rise of Totalitarian Democracy (Boston, 1952), pp. 21–22.

7. J.J. Rousseau, Émile, ou l'éducation, Oeuvres complètes (Paris, 1959), 4:663. "This [masturbation] is one of the principle causes of the degeneration of the race in the cities. Young men, weakened early in life remain small, weak, poorly built, aged, instead of

grown, like the vine which bearing fruit in the spring languishes and dies before autumn." *Émile*, 4:496. For Rousseau's own penchant for "ce dangereux supplément qui trompe la nature" see his *Confessions, Oeuvres complètes* (Paris, 1959), 1:109.

8. J.J. Rousseau, *Discours sur l'inégalité, Oeuvres complètes* (Paris, 1959) 3:633.

9. Charles Eynard, *Tissot*, (Paris, 1839), p. 88.

10. J.J. Rousseau, *Correspondance complète*, ed. R.A. Leigh (Madison, Wisconsin, 1970) 12:82. See also A. François, "Rousseau et Tissot," *Annales de la société Jean-Jacques Rousseau* (1911) 7:19–40 and François Jost, *Jean-Jacques Rousseau, Suisse* (Fribourg, 1961) 1:341–342.

11. From d'Holbach's *System of Nature* cited by W.H. Wickwar, *Baron d'Holbach: A Prelude to the French Revolution*, 2nd ed. (New York, 1968) p. 164.

12. Moreover, the physician was to replace the priest as the instructor in good behavior. Diderot declared, "Ask the doctor . . . Is your child voluptuous? Make him hunt all day and at night, have him drink a concoction of nenuphar; that is worth more than a chapter of Seneca." J. Assezat, ed., *Réfutation de l'ouvrage d'Helvétius* in *Oeuvres complètes* (Paris, 1875), 2:283

13. *Dictionnaire philosophique* (Paris, 1832), 3:196–197.

14. On Dutoit-Mambrini see Jules Chavannes, *Jean-Philippe Dutoit* (Lausanne, 1865).

15. Dutoit-Mambrini, *L'Onanisme* (Lausanne, 1760, p. 42.

16. Ibid., pp. 59–60.

17. Ibid., p. 60.

18. Ibid., p. 61.

19. See, for example, *La Religieuse* (Paris, 1795) and *Le Rêve d'Alembert* (Paris, 1830).

20. An English admirer of Tissot was John Wesley who described *Avis au people* as the most useful medical text to appear in the century and published extracts of the work in his own health manual. See A. Wesley Hall, *John Wesley Among the Physicians: A Study of Eighteenth Century Medicine* (London, 1958), pp. 54–82.

21. Tissot, *Avis au people* (Lausanne, 1763), pp. 7–8.

22. Ibid., p. 9.

23. Moheau (a *nom de plume*), *Recherches et considérations sur la population*, 2:104. Cf. 1:144. Le Chevalier de Cerfol denounced contraception as not only immoral and antisocial but psychologically harmful; S.N.H. Linguet declared that sexual excesses led to sterility. See J.J. Spengler, *Economie et population: Les Doctrines françaises avant 1800* (Paris, 1954) pp. 312, 370. Mirabeau declared: "Nature shudders at the means luxury suggests to avoid the embarrassment of a numerous family." *L'Ami des hommes* (Paris, 1755), part I, Chapter VII and see also part II, Chapter VII.

24. C.F. Volney, *Catéchisme du citoyen français, Oeuvres complètes* (Paris, 1821), 1:280–281. That the attack on clerical celibacy as a cause of immorality and depopulation was not to be shortlived can be gauged by a glance at such works as M. Blanchet, *Les Funestes effets de la vertu de chasteté dans les prêtres* (Paris, 1790); F.E. Fodéré, *Essai historique et moral sur la pauvreté des nations* (Paris, 1825).

25. Volney, *Catéchisme*, 1:282.

26. Millot and Coffin-Rosny, *Le Nestor français*, 1:157–158, and see also Mme. H. Azais, *Des Compensations dans les destinées humaines* (Paris, 1810).

27. Millot and Coffin-Rosny, *Le Nestor français*, 2:129.

28. Ibid., 3:100. The authors declared that such an action constituted the crime of *lèse-nation*.

29. The Empire did see one of the first published apologies of contraception in Etienne de

Sénancour, *De l'amour* (Paris, 1806), pp. 170–173. See also pp. 412–417 for Sénancour's critique of both Rousseau's antifeminism and the general eighteenth-century fear of depopulation.

30. See also J.L. Alibert, *Physiologie des passions* (Paris, 1826) and M. Fournier-Verneuil, *Paris: Tableau moral et physiologique* (Paris, 1826).

31. Lallemand, *Des Pertes séminales involuntaires*, 3:475, 476.

32. The claim that the decadence of the East was caused by sexual intemperance had already been made in the nineteenth century by J.J. Virey, *Hygiène philosophique* (Paris, 1828), 2:74. The belief that the West had to retain its sexual purity if it was to carry out its imperialistic calling was shared by Baden-Powell, who insisted on referring to the penis as the "racial organ." See Robert H. MacDonald, "The Frightful Consequences of Onanism: Notes on the History of a Delusion," *Journal of the History of Ideas* 28 (1967), 430.

33. Raspail, *Histoire naturelle de la santé et de la maladie*, (Paris, 1843), 2:604ff.

34. J.B.D. Demeaux, *Mémoire sur l'onanisme* (Paris, 1857), pp. 18–19.

35. For similar fixations see Debourge de Rollot, *Le Mémento du père de famille* (Paris, 1860), p. 5.

36. François Quesnay, *Questions intéressantes sur la population, l'agriculture et le commerce* in Institut National d'Etudes Démographique, *François Quesnay et la physiocratie* (Paris, 1968), p. 664.

37. For an early plea for moral restraint on the part of workers see Charles Dunoyer, *Mémoire à consulter sur quelques-unes des principales questions que la révolution de Juillet a fait naitre* (Paris, 1835), p. 176. One should note that even a Catholic economist like Alban Villeneuve-Bargemont who was opposed to birth control could recommend late marriages in *Economie politique Chrétienne* (Paris, 1834), 3 vol.

38. Joseph Garnier, *Journal des économistes* 38 (1863), 148–155; cf. 9 (1880), 241–248. See also J.J. Spengler, *France Faces Depopulation* (Durham, N.C., 1938), pp. 50ff and "French Population Theory Since 1800," *Journal of Political Economy* 44 (1936), 577—631, 743—766.

39. P.J.C. Debreyne, *Essai sur la théologie morale* (Paris, 1846), vi, 54. See also L.E. Bautain, *Philosophie morale* (Paris, 1842), 1:232–235.

40. A.M. Barthélemy stated quite categorically that Tissot's works aroused as much as they frightened readers: *Syphilis* (Paris, 1840), p. iv.

41. Balzac's *Médecin de campagne* vividly documents the doctor's replacement of the priest as a moral force in the countryside. Sixty-three of the characters in the *Comédie humaine* are involved with medicine in some way. See G. Pradalie, *Balzac historien* (Paris, 1955), pp. 68—69. Auguste Comte declared that "Civilization . . . requires that the function of the physician be more and more absorbed into the office of the priest, instead of sanctioning the ever widening divergence of the two, which was applicable only to the Western transition." *System of Positive Polity*, trans. Richard Congreve (London, 1877), 4:247. See also Georges Audiffret, *Appel aux médecins* (Paris, 1862).

42. See, for example, Philippe Ariès in Bergues, *La Prévention des naissances*, pp. 311–327.

43. Honoré de Balzac, *Mémoires de deux jeunes mariées: Oeuvres complètes* (Paris, 1869), 1:202.

44. A. Bazin, *L'époque sans nom: Esquisse de Paris, 1830–1833* (Paris, 1833) 1:40.

45. Edmond About, *Maître Pierre* (Paris, 1858), p. 219.

46. R. Bruckner, *Les Intimes* (Paris, 1831), 3:388.

CHAPTER FIVE

1. Georges Sorel, *Matériaux d'une théorie du prolétariat* (Paris, 1919), p. 196. For the purposes of this chapter no stringent definition of socialism is necessary; the term "the left" will be used to mean the socialist left.
2. J.P. Dutoit-Mambrini, *L'Onanisme ou discours philosophiques et moral sur la luxure artificielle & sur tous les crimes relatifs* (Lausanne, 1760), p. 60.
3. Moheau, *Recherches et considérations sur la population de la France* (Paris, 1778), 2:102.
4. Père Féline, *Catéchisme des gens mariés* (Paris, 1880), p. 9.
5. Dr. A. Mayer, *Des Rapports conjugaux* (Paris, 1857), p. 144.
6. M. Guyau, *L'Irréligion de l'avenir* (Paris, 1887), pp. 282–82.
7. Charles Gide, "Le dépeuplement de la France", *La Revue hebdomadaire* 19 (8 May 1909), 143 (the addenda are Gide's).
8. J.J. Spengler, *France Faces Depopulation* (Durham, 1938) and "French Population Theory Since 1800," *Journal of Political Economy* 44 (1936): 577–631; René Goddard, *Histoire des doctrines de la population* (Paris, 1923); Francesco Nitti, *Population and the Social System* (London, 1894).
9. J.J. Rousseau, *Du contrat social* (Amsterdam, 1762), p. 119.
10. François-Noël Babeuf, *Du système de dépopulation* (Paris, an III), p. 35. Though this passage is taken from his response to the reputed Jacobin plot to depopulate France it is representative of Babeuf's thinking. The association of depopulation with the excesses of the Terror was a theme later popularized by Taine.
11. T.R. Malthus, *An Essay on the Principles of Population* (London, 1803), p. 531.
12. Frank E. Manuel, *The New World of Henri Saint-Simon* (Cambridge, Mass., 1965), pp. 227–28.
13. A. Comte, *Cours de philosophie positive* (Paris, 1842), 4:644ff. Sismonde de Sismondi could be included here as a left-leaning liberal critical of Malthus; see his *Nouveaux principes d'économie politique* (Paris, 1819), 2:248ff. and *Etudes sur l'économie politique* (Paris, 1837), 1:130; 2:266ff.
14. Philippe-Michel Buonarroti, *Conspiration pour l'égalité* (Paris, 1828), p. 120.
15. Étienne Cabet, *Voyage en Icarie* (Paris, 1842), p. 121.
16. P.J. Proudhon, *Système des contradictions économiques ou, philosophie de la misère*, (Paris, 1846), 2:449. At about the same time Proudhon wrote to an economist friend; "All that has been written on this subject inspires in me a profound disgust: it is inexpressibly pitiful. So I, like you, Sir, am a Malthusian; but an ultra-Malthusian, which is to say that reliance must be exclusively on *abstinence* in this matter of population. . . . As to the future, I believe in *mores* very different from ours; in a spirituality in love such as Plato advanced, and of which Christianity has given us more than one example. I regard our present lasciviousness as wholly unnatural; all that parade of tenderness, however honourable and delicate; all those burning expressions, too, on the subject of women, which modern writing is full of, seem to me to be an expression of disordered erotic excitement rather than a symptom of legitimate tendencies. . . . " Cited by Edward Hyams, *Pierre-Joseph Proudhon; His Revolutionary Life, Mind, and Works* (London, 1979), p. 64.
17. Pierre Leroux, *Malthus et les économistes* (Paris, 1849), pp. 104–105.
18. Ibid., p. 104. Leroux was apparently referring to Marcus (a *nom de plume*), *An Essay on Populousness* (London, 1838) not realizing that it was a Swiftian attack on, not a defense of, infanticide.

19. The socialist's faith in nature mirrored the Catholic's faith in the Creator, e.g., Père
    Féline, Catéchisme, pp. 41–42.

20. Proudhon, Système des contradictions, 2:453, 456; Charles Loudon, The Equilibrium of
    Population and Sustenance Demonstrated (London, 1836).

21. Système des contradictions, 2:455.

22. Ibid., 2:477.

23. Cf. T. Dézamy, Code de la communauté (Paris, 1842), p. 193.

24. Louis Blanc, Organization du travail (Paris, 1848), pp. 152–53. Blanc came close to
    saying, as had the conservative Catholic H.A. Frégier, that only the sober artisan would
    have the self-control necessary to practice coitus interruptus. Frégier also made the
    interesting point that the self-centered artisan who adopted the practice would soon
    shed the traditional lower-class sympathy for unwed mothers and illegitimate children:
    Des classes dangereuses de la population dans les grandes villes (Paris, 1840)
    1:326–35.

25. Louis-Auguste Blanqui, Critique sociale (Paris, 1885), 1:143–44.

26. For similar arguments on food and falling birth rates see Charles Fourier, Le Nouveau
    Monde industriel in Oeuvres (Paris, 1841–45), 4:337ff. and from the other side of the
    Channel, Thomas Doubleday, The True Law of Population (London, 1842), p. 275.

27. Morelly, Code de la nature (Paris, 1910), p. 99.

28. J.J. Rousseau, Émile ou de l'éducation in Oeuvres complètes (Paris, 1971), 3:25.

29. Cited by Philippe-Michel Buonarroti, Système politique (Paris, 1842), pp. 49–50.
    Babeuf was given to the use of Samson and Delilah imagery.

30. Buonarroti, Conspiration pour l'égalité, 1:282–83.

31. Cabet, Icarie (Paris, 1842) pp. 40 and 122. On the idea of systematic procreation
    reserved for the best physical and intellectual specimens cf. Auguste Comte, Système
    de politique positive (Paris, 1851), 4:278.

32. For example, George Lichtheim, The Origins of Socialism (London, 1969), p. 244 and
    F. Manuel, The Prophets of Paris (Cambridge, Mass., 1962), p. 157.

33. S. Charléty, Enfantin (Paris, 1930); Michel Chevalier, ed., Religion saint-simonienne
    (Paris, 1832), pp. 176–81; Mme. de Casamajor (Emile Barrault), Pathologie du
    mariage (Paris, 1847).

34. Comte was basically a conservative but deserves attention here because many of his
    ideas were shared by writers on the left. The fourth part of volume one of Système de
    politique positive was devoted to the Influence féminine de positivisme. See also L.M.
    Ferré, Féminisme et positivisme (Paris, 1938).

35. Comte, Politique positive, 1:210; 4:68–69, 276–78. The climax of this process was,
    logically enough, virgin birth. Polygamy had been displaced by monogamy; now
    maternity was to be reconciled with virginity! Ibid., 4:69, 278.

36. P.J. Proudhon, De la justice dans la révolution et dans l'église (Paris, 1858), 3:375.

37. P.J. Proudhon, La Pornocratie ou les femmes dans les temps modernes (Paris, 1875),
    p. 181.

38. Proudhon, La Pornocratie, pp. 262–263. On the fear of female licentiousness see
    Alphonse Esquiros, Paris ou les sciences, les institutions et les moeurs au XIXᵉ siècle
    (Paris, 1847), 2:355; and compare Proudhon's baleful warnings to Flaubert's
    admonishment of Ernest Feydau: "But be careful not to injure your intelligence in
    relationships with ladies. You will lose your genius at the end of a womb . . . Keep your
    priapism for style, f. . .your inkpot, calm yourself with meat, and be convinced, as Tissot
    (of Geneva) said (Traité de l'onanie, page 72, see the engraving), that the loss of one

ounce of sperm is more fatiguing than that of three liters of blood." *Correspondance* (Paris, 1929), 4:312.

39. Jules Michelet, *L'Amour* (Paris, 1889), p. 52.
40. Proudhon, *La Pornocratie*, p. 227.
41. But see Marguerite Thibert, *Le Féminisme dans le socialisme française de 1830 à 1850* (Paris, 1926).
42. François Vidal, *De la répartition des richesses* (Paris, 1846), p. 285; cf. Ernest Legouvé, *Histoire morale des femmes* (Paris, 1849), p. 332.
43. Saint-Simon's statement that the happy man was the working man typified this outlook: *Introduction aux travaux scientifiques de XIXe siècle*, in *Oeuvres* (Paris, 1839), 1:220ff.
44. Leroux, *Malthus et les économistes*, p. 183. Proudhon declared: "*Onanism* has as its corollary *bestiality*. It's curious; conjugal onanism has been proposed by the defenders of human exploitation in order to serve as a brake on the population: as if the bestiality of economics was sanctioned by the bestiality of love." *De la justice*, 3:485.
45. P.J.B. Buchez and U. Trélat, *Précis élémentaire d'hygiène* (Paris, 1825), p. 219.
46. Buchez, *Précis*, p. 220.
47. Proudhon, *Système de contradictions*, 2:480.
48. Ibid., 2:496.
49. Georges Sorel, *Matériaux d'une théorie du prolétariat* (Paris, 1919), p. 198.
50. Ibid., p. 199. Compare Babeuf's statement of a hundred years earlier: "Les moeurs étant les garantes des Républiques parce que celles-ci basent sur les vertus, c'est des institutions morales que dépend la perfection ou la perversion de l'esprit républicain." *Le Tribune du peuple* 28 (Paris, n.d.), 240.
51. Alfred Naquet, *L'Humanité et la patrie* (Paris, 1901), p. 243.
52. Dr. Alexandre Picon, *Aperçu sur les principales causes de la dépopulation* (Paris, 1888), p. 9. The information on the size of doctors' families is provided by Dr. Minime (Dr. Auguste Lutaud), *Le Néo-Malthisanisme* (Paris, 1891), p. 14.

CHAPTER SIX

1. Gabriel Giroud, *Paul Robin* (Paris, 1937), pp. 24–25.
2. On Robin's early life see Giroud, *Robin*, pp. 11–25.
3. See Rosanna Ledbetter, *A History of the Malthusian League, 1877–1927* (Columbus, Ohio, 1976) and Angus McLaren, *Birth Control in Nineteenth Century England* (London, 1978), pp. 107–113.
4. James Guillaume, *L'Internationale* (Paris, 1905), 4:223; Giroud, *Robin*, p. 22–25.
5. On Cempuis see Gabriel Giroud, *Cempuis* (Paris, 1900) and Angus McLaren, "Revolution and Education in Late Nineteenth Century France: The Early Career of Paul Robin," *History of Education Quarterly*, 21 (1981), pp. 317–335.
6. *National Reformer* (20 July 1884), p. 58; *Malthusian* (July 1884), p. 538; (October 1893), p. 73; (May 1895), p. 35.
7. *Malthusian* (July 1895), pp. 50–51; Giroud, *Robin*, p. 88.
8. *.Malthusian* (June 1896), p. 45.
9. *Le Figaro* (13 January 1897), p. 1; *Le Temps* (11 January 1897), p. 1; *La République française* (15 January 1897), p. 1.
10. On Robin's account of the events of 1897 see *Régénération* (April 1900) and (January 1903). See also the special flyer of the summer of 1897 put out by *Régénération* in

which it was asserted that the Darlan-Béranger bill against outrages against morality was aimed at the Ligue.

11. *Malthusian* (October 1898), p. 75. Robin cited Leygoens, Cornely, Lombelins, and Bertillon as responsible for his persecution. See also Giroud, *Robin*, pp. 233–234. See also *Le Gaulois* (11 January 1897), p. 1.

12. Robin reported in *Régénération* (April 1908): "I saw in the Antipodes ingenious housewives who made for themselves a derisory price an object having the same efficacy as the best brands of pessaries, ovules, cones. . . . " Bickerton — apparently influenced by Max Nordau — had organized a curious commune of about thirty people living in tar paper shacks and producing fireworks. See R.M. Burdon, *Scholar Errant: A Biography of A.W. Bickerton* (Christchurch, 1956), pp. 69–70; see also *Malthusian* (April 1899), pp. 26, 36–37; (June 1899), p. 42; (July 1899), p. 50.

13. It was reported in 1904 that the Ligue had a thousand subscribers and about twenty sections. See *Malthusian* (February 1904), p. 9.

14. See, for example, Joseph Droz, *Economie politique ou, principes de la science des richesses* (Paris, 1854), pp. 261–268.

15. See, for example, Charles Denoyer, *Mémoire à consulter sur quelque-unes des principales questions que la revolution de Juillet a fait naître* (Paris, 1835), p. 176. and on the general issue J.J. Spengler, *France Faces Depopulation* (Durham, 1938), pp. 141–142.

16. See, for example, Edmond Desfossé, *Décroissance de la population en France* (Paris, 1869).

17. J.J. Rapet, *Manuel de morale et d'économie politique à l'usage des classes ouvrières* (Paris, 1853), pp. 461–462; see also the classic scene of middle-class contempt for workers' fecundity in Emile Zola, *Germinal* (Paris, 1885).

18. McLaren, *Birth Control*, pp. 51–56.

19. Robert Dale Owen, *Moral Physiology* (New York, 1830), pp. 60–61.

20. Charles R. Drysdale, "La Doctrine de Malthus," *Gazette médicale de Paris* 7 (1878), pp. 53–532. See also *National Reformer* (25 August 1878), pp. 113–114. Drysdale was indefatigable in his attempts to woo the French. He defended Malthusian doctrines at the 1895 Paris Medical Congress (and later asserted that Bertillon *fils* established the Alliance nationale contre la dépopulation as a response), he assisted at the founding of Robin's Ligue in 1896, and he attended the International Malthusian Conference in Paris in 1900.

21. A. Talandier was also an honorary vice-president of Bradlaugh's Secular Society; see *National Reformer* (1878); *Malthusian* (October 1879), p. 69; (April 1883), p. 408.

22. On French views of the Malthusian League see "La Ligue Malthusienne: son origine et son histoire," *Journal des économistes* 11 (1880), 241–248; Pierre Mille, "Le Néo-Malthusienne en Angleterre," *Revue des deux mondes* 108 (15 December 1891), 911–928. It might be noted that birth control was so associated with English economics in French minds that the verb "malthusianiser" was coined to describe the practice.

23. Paul Robin, *Malthus et les néo-Malthusiens* (Paris, 1905), p. 3.

24. See McLaren, "Paul Robin," passim.

25. G. Vacher de Lapouge, *Les sélections sociales* (Paris, 1896).

26. Reprinted as Dr. Minime, *Le Néo-Malthusianisme: lettre à M. Max Hausmeister* (Paris, 1891). See Drysdale's warm review in *Malthusian* (January 1892), pp. 4–5.

27. See Robin's speech reported in *Bulletin de la société d'anthropologie de Paris* 7 (1896), 139–40, 143, 210–212, 224; and also *Régénération* (November 1905).

28. *Malthusian* (April 1896) pp. 25–27; *Régénération* (December 1896), p. 3.

29. See Michael Freeden, "Eugenics and Progressive Thought: A Study in Ideological Affinity," *Historical Journal* 22 (1979), 645–672.

30. See *Malthusian* (August 1900); *Régénération* (May, 1902); Giroud, *Robin*, p. 224.

31. Bitterly disappointed by doctors' indifference to birth control, Robin attacked them for preferring to deal with the symptoms of overpopulation such as tuberculosis and alcoholism and warmly reviewed the antimedical tract of Charles Soller and Louis Gastine, *Défends ton peau contre ton médecine* (Paris, 1902). See *Régénération* (May 1902).

32. T.R. Malthus, *An Essay on the Principles of Population* (London, 1798), p. 154.

33. Antoine-Nicholas de Condorcet, *Esquisse d'un tableau historique des progrès de l'esprit humain*, ed. O.H. Prior (Paris, 1933), pp. 222–23.

34. Etienne de Sénancour, *De l'amour*, 3rd ed. (Paris, 1834), 1:332.

35. Sénancour, *De l'amour*, 2nd ed. (Paris, 1808), pp. 41, 146.

36. Sénancour specifically defended the unmarried woman's right to contraception: *De l'amour* (1808), p. 145; (1834), 1:245.

37. Charles Fourier, *Passions of the Human* cited by Spengler, *France*, p. 72.

38. For denunciations of Fourier see Proudhon, *Système des contradictions*, 2:451–55 and Sorel, *Matériaux d'une théorie*, p. 196.

39. Charles Fourier, *Le Nouveau Monde industriel*, in *Oeuvres* (Paris, 1841–45), 4:337ff. Moreover, Fourier believed that the land could support a larger population if organized in horticultural communities; he drew support for his argument from M. Herrenschwand, *De l'économie politique moderne; discours fondamental sur la population* (London, 1786).

40. Charles Fourier, *Duperies des détracteurs; Secte Owen*, in *Oeuvres*, 4:154–155.

41. Charles Fourier, *Le Nouveau Monde amoureux*, in *Théorie des quatres mouvements et des destinées générales* (Paris, 1967), pp. 245–314. Fourier's followers tended to downplay his interest in sex, e.g., Victor Hennequin, *Les Amours au phalanstère* (Paris, 1849). It is of interest to note, however, that Dr. A. Mayer, one of the first doctors to publicly defend contraception, hailed Fourier as "un grand génie moderne." *Des Rapports conjugaux* (Paris, 1849), p. 106.

42. Giroud, *Robin*, p. 209.

43. Ibid., p. 214.

44. Ibid., p. 214.

45. *Régénération* (December 1896), p. 1.

46. Robin, *Le Néo-Malthusianisme*, pp. 7–10; and see also Paul Robin, "La Question de néo-Malthusianisme," *Revue de morale sociale* (1903), pp. 202–203.

47. Robin went so far in his sex radicalism as to attempt to improve the lot of prostitutes — not by "rescuing them — but by organizing them." He believed that in the long run birth control by permitting greater sexual freedom would put an end to prostitution; in the short run he saw prostitutes fulfilling an unfortunately necessary role though one in which they risked their health and indeed their lives. Accordingly the task was to protect as much as possible women who were as virtuous as many wives, not by police regulation which only led to the appearance of pimps and extortion, but by the unionization of the prostitutes for their own self-defense. Robin advanced his views in *Propos d'une fille* but his hopes of establishing a *Ligue anti-esclavage* and a journal, *Le Cri de filles*, came to nothing because of police hostility. See Giroud, *Robin*, pp. 164–165.

48. Paul Robin, *Population et prudence procréatrice* (Paris, 1892), p. 4.

49. Ibid., p. 6.

50. Robin to Vandervelde, 25 January 1903, cited in *Giroud*, Robin, p. 137. See also *Régénération* (July 1902); (April 1903).

51. On the meeting see *Malthusian* (September 1900); *Régénération* (January 1901). Other French activists included Victor Dave, Gilbert Lenoir, M. Myries, M. Petit, Botdy, and Bariol. *Régénération* also noted the propaganda campaigns outside of France such as those of the Drysdales in England and Ida Craddock, Emma Goldman, and Moses Harmon in America. Quebec, because of its high birth rate was cited frequently as a negative example of the dangers of overpopulation. The report of land being given by the provincial government to large French-Canadian families elicited the response, "Ca, c'est plutôt bébête." For other references to "lapinisme canadien" see *Régénération* (July 1907) and *Génération consciente* (October 1910).

52. Roussel made a first appearance in April 1903, Humbert in March 1903 with an article on "la grève de ventre," and Desplanques in June 1903 with an essay "Ayez peu d'enfants" in which he declared that workers needed "les coudes franches pour la lutte."

53. On prosecutions see *Régénération* (May 1901), (April 1906); *Génération consciente* (15 July 1908); *Malthusian* (September 1900), p. 68.

54. See a report of the meeting in *Régénération* (August 1903). The syndicalist press also spread word of Robin's activities. *Régénération* listed as papers friendly to the cause and willing to reprint propaganda: *L'Ouvrier coiffeur, Réveil des mécaniciens, Le Combat de Levallois-Clichy, Le Relieur, L'Ouvrier métallurgiste, L'Ouvrier syndiqué* (Marseilles), *L'Emancipation* (Toulon), *Réveil syndical* (Lens), *Voix du peuple, Réveil de l'esclave, L'Idée socialiste* (Lyon), *Le Jura socialiste, Le Progrès* (Le Havre), *L'Insurgé* (Liege), *Le Travailleur syndiqué* (Montpellier), *L'Action ouvrière* (Bordeaux), *Le Combat* (Bordeaux), *Petit république* (Paris), *L'Action* (Paris), *Cri de quartier* (Paris), *La Cravache* (Rheims).

55. See *Régénération* (December 1896). In 1905 the Ligue also began to distribute a series of gummed propaganda labels to be stuck on walls. A typical one read:

> L'Avortement est dangereux
> La prévention de la grossesse
> est facile et sans danger
> AYONS PEU D'ENFANTS

56. The concern for the expense of contraceptives was noted in a cartoon of Alphonse Lévy showing a working woman looking at a shop window display of preventives and exclaiming, "Ca, c'est trop cher pour moi." *Régénération* (February, 1902).

57. *Régénération* (April 1908). In *Controverse sur le néo-Malthusianisme* (1905) Robin listed the practitioners to be consulted but warned, "Requests for abortion will not be replied to." Those listed included Dr. Adrien Meslier, Dr. J. Darricarrère, Marot (*herboriste*), Mme. H. Piens (*sage-femme*), M. et Mme. Eugène Humbert, Mme. Petit (*sage-femme*), and other "pharmaciens" and "aide-pharmaciens."

58. Dr. Brennus, *Amour et securité* (Paris, 1906); Dr. Brennus, *Histoire du célèbre ouvrage amour et securité* (Paris, 1895).

59. Giroud, *Robin*, pp. 253–260.

60. *Le Malthusien* (November—December 1908). In November 1910 Robin was referred to as "le vieux satyr" in the *Malthusien* because of his purported views on the need for sexual initiation of the young and the efficacy of extended nursing as a means to avoid conception.

61. *Le Malthusien* (October 1910), (September 1912).

62. *Le Malthusien* (April, June 1912), (March 1913).

63. Jeanne Humbert, *Eugène Humbert: La vie et l'oeuvre d'un néo-malthusian* (Paris, 1947).

64. Those who rallied to *Génération consciente*'s platform included such left-wing personalities as Edouard Ganche, "Germinal," Dr. Meslier, Eugène Lericolais, Albert Lecomte, and Thérèse Clément, widow of the poet, J.B. Clément.

65. It should also be noted that *Génération consciente* chose to ignore the activities of the conservative English Malthusian League but reported the actions of the Belgian, Swiss, and German movements.

66. *Génération consciente* (15 April 1908).

67. *Génération consciente* (1 March 1909).

68. On prosecutions see *Génération consciente* (1 March 1909), (December 1909), (15 November 1908); *Le Malthusian* (January 1913), (February 1913). While Humbert was in jail the paper was edited by Robin's son-in-law, Gabriel Giroud.

69. *Génération consciente* (May 1910).

70. *Génération consciente* (15 September 1908), (February 1910), (June 1912).

71. On Dr. Fernand Mascaux see D.V. Glass, *Population Policies and Movements in Europe* (London, 1967), p. 444 and Ph. Van Praag, "The Development of Neo-Malthusianism in Flanders," *Population Studies* 32 (1978), 467–480.

72. *Génération consciente* (May 1912), (April 1914).

73. *Génération consciente* (September 1910).

CHAPTER SEVEN

1. *Malthusian* (October, 1920).

2. Jacques Freymond, ed., *La première internationale* (Geneva, 1962), 1:217–218.

3. Freymond, *Internationale*, pp. 220–221.

4. On Germany see R.P. Neuman, "Working-Class Birth Control in Wilhemine Germany," *Comparative Studies in Society and History* 20 (1978):408–428.

5. V.I. Lenin, *Collected Works* (Moscow, 1963), 19:237; see also Jean Freville, *La Femme et le communisme* (Paris, 1951), p. 134.

6. On Jaurès see Harvey Goldberg, *The Life of Jean Jaurès* (Madison, 1962), and *Génération consciente*, (15 September 1908); and on Blum see William Logue, *Léon Blum: The Formative Years: 1872–1914* (De Kalb, Illinois, 1973) and *Régénération*, (July 1907), p. 267.

7. Désiré Descamps, "Le Problème de la dépopulation," *Revue socialiste* 24 (1896), 257–285. Robin had submitted articles on fertility control to the *Revue socialiste* in 1890 and 1891 but they were rejected by Benoît Malon on the grounds that their appearance would cause an uproar in the socialist camp. See Gabriel Giroud, *Paul Robin* (Paris, 1937), p. 209.

8. Désiré Descamps, "Le Problème de l'amour," *Revue socialiste* 25 (1897), 641–657; 26 (1897), 18–46. See also Aline Valette and M. Bonnier, *Socialisme et sexualisme* (Paris, 1893) and Dr. Lux on "Le Malthusianisme bourgeois" in *L'Intransigent* (10 February 1885).

9. Dr. Pax Salvat, *La Dépopulation de la France* (Paris, 1903), p. 43. Pax Salvat's true identity is unknown.

10. Henri Dagan, "Réponse aux néo-malthusiens," L'Oeuvre nouvelle, (1903–1904), p. 128. See also the debate in Le Libertaire in 1904 and 1905.

11. Dagan, "Réponse," p. 133.

12. Ibid., p. 136.

13. Dr. Oguse, "Socialisme et néo-malthusianisme," Revue socialiste 46 (1907), 97–124. To the question of whether birth control was good inasmuch as it spared women the pain of unwanted pregnancies Oguse insultingly responded, asking, "But constipation is also a great misery and prevents some people from listening to reason; why not create a league for the regeneration of humanity by the use of laxatives?" (p. 123).

14. Cited in Roger H. Guerrand, La Libre Maternité, 1896–1969 (Paris, 1971), p. 58 and see also André Armengaud, "Mouvement ouvrier et néo-malthusianisme au début du 20e siècle," Annales de démographie historique (1966), 7–21.

15. Robert Hertz, Socialisme et dépopulation: Les cahiers du Socialiste, no. 10 (Paris, 1910), p. 16.

16. Hertz, Socialisme, p. 17. Although the antimilitarist Henri Barbusse attended an international neo-Malthusian conference in 1925, he also had printed in his journal that same year an article by Jean Montreuil that echoed Hertz in asserting that socialists had to choose between a poor, pure, numerous working class and a "class of embourgeoised foremen, controlling their fertility, and overseeing millions of yellow and black workers." Clarté (1925), p. 159.

17. Revue socialiste 53 (1911), 475–476.

18. See Paul Lafargue, La Question de la femme (Paris, 1904), pp. 22–24; Jules Guesde, Essai de catéchisme socialiste (Paris, 1878), pp. 93–98. On the hostility of the Communist Party to birth control between the wars, see Jean Freville, La Misère et le nombre: l'épouvantail malthusien (Paris, 1956); François Delpa, "Les Communistes français et la sexualité, 1932–1938," Mouvement sociale 91 (1975), 121–152.

19. Cited by Jean Maitron, Histoire du mouvement anarchiste en France, 1880–1914, (Paris, 1951), pp. 38–39.

20. Guillaume to Paul Robin, cited by Giroud, Robin, p. 202.

21. Kropotkin to Robin, cited by Giroud, Robin, p. 202 and see also Revue de morale sociale (1903), p. 353, and see also Peter Kropotkin, Fields, Factories and Workshops (London, 1899), pp. 103–126; George Woodcock and Ivan Avakumovic, The Anarchist Prince: A Biographical Study of Peter Kropotkin (London, 1950) pp. 148–149.

22. Jean Grave, La Société future (Paris, 1895), p. 356; and on Robin see Mireille Delfau, Jean Grave: Quarante ans de propagande anarchiste (Paris, 1973), pp. 342–343, and Régénération (August 1903), p. 195.

23. See Marie Fleming, The Anarchist Way to Socialism: Elisée Reclus and Nineteenth Century European Anarchism (London, 1979), pp. 231, 237.

24. See Madeleine Vernet, Le Libertaire (8–15 September 1907), and see for similar views Dr. Pierrot, Les Temps nouveaux (April 1911). Vernet did share Robin's concern for the education of working-class children. See her Les Sans-familles du proletariat organisé (Epone, 1911). On feminists and birth control, see chapter ten.

25. Victor Serge, Memoirs of a Revolutionary, 1901–1948 (Oxford, 1963), pp. 12–22; on Italy see Paulo Mantegazza, Igiene dell'amore (Florence, 1903); G. Pini and D. Susmel, Mussolini (Florence, 1953), 1:127–128 and Laura Fermi, Mussolini (Chicago, 1961), p. 65; on Spain see Giroud, Robin, p. 239. Jeanne Humbert asserted that before the war even Sun-Yat-Sen came to Paris seeking birth control information from Eugène Humbert. See Jeanne Humbert, Eugène Humbert: la vie et l'oeuvre d'un néo-malthusien (Paris, 1948), p. 81.

26. See, for example, André Lorulot and Abbé J. Viollet, *L'Église et l'amour* (Paris, 1929).
27. Jean Bidegrain, *Le Grand Orient de France* (Paris, 1905), pp. 200–214. Given the fact that his book was published by the "Libraire antisémite" Bidegrain's point of view is made fairly clear.
28. Maurice Dommanget, *La Chevalerie du travail français, 1893–1911* (Paris, 1967), pp. 240–246, 259–266, 293–296, 540.
29. Alfred Naquet, *Autobiographie* (Paris, 1939) and A. Naquet and G. Hardy, *Néo-malthusianisme et socialisme* (Paris, 1910). See also Victor Ernest, *Socialisme et néo-malthusianisme* (Paris, n.d.), distributed by *Génération consciente*.
30. *Journal des débats* (4 April 1911), p. 1.
31. Sébastien Faure, *Le Problème de la dépopulation (Paris, 1908) and Défendons-nous: Pour les néo-Malthusianisme contre l'immoralité des "moralistes."* (Paris, 1910). See also on Faure, Jean Finot, *Préjugé et problème des sexes* (Paris, 1913), p. 459.
32. See also Un Malthusien (a *nom de plume*), *La Grève de l'amour* (Paris, 1891); Fernand Kolney, *La Grève des ventres* (Paris, 1910), Emile Chapelier, *Ayons peu d'enfants* (Paris, n.d.), and Frank Sutor [Cordonnier], *Génération consciente* (Paris, n.d.).
33. See G. Hardy, *Moyens d'éviter la grossesse* (Paris, 1908) and *La Loi de Malthus* (Paris, 1909). See also Giroud's account of the birth control campaign in France in *Report of the Fifth Neo-Malthusian and Birth Control Conference* (London, 1922), pp. 23–25.
34. See E. Armand, *sa vie, sa pensée, son oeuvre* (Paris, 1964).
35. Devaldès also translated into French C.L. James, *Malthus et l'anarchisme* (Paris, 1910). See also Hem Day, ed., *Un en-dehors: Manuel Devaldès, 1875–1956: Les Cahiers pensée et action* (1957), pp. 7–8.
36. See, for example, André Lorulot, *Crime et société: essai de criminologie sociale* (Paris, 1922).
37. Ernest Tarbouriech, *La Cité future: essai d'une utopie scientifique* (Paris, 1902), pp. 298–307 and see also *Régénération* (September 1902), p. 103. For a contemporary work of similar bent see Paulo Mantegazza, *L'Anno 3000* (Florence, 1897).
38. Remy de Gourmont, *Dialogue des amateurs sur les choses de temps,* (1897) 1:98; (1905–1907) 4:52. Gourmont was to reveal his continuing interest in sex reforms by arranging for the translation of Havelock Ellis's works and writing his own *Physique de l'amour: essai sur l'instinct sexuel* (Paris, 1912). The writings of Paul Adam and Victor Marguerite were also frequently cited by contemporaries as containing implicit defenses of the woman's right to control her own body.
39. *Le Canard sauvage* 16 (5–11 July 1913).
40. *L'Assiette au beurre* (4 October 1902), (8 November 1902), (27 August 1904), (13 April 1907).
41. Léon Frapie, *La Maternelle* (Paris, 1905), p. 266.
42. Ferri-Pisani, *Sterilité* (Paris, 1906), p. 96. For an overview of the literature dealing with questions of sexuality, see Guy de Téramond, *L'Adoration perpetuelle* (Paris, 1902).

CHAPTER EIGHT

1. Paul Cauwès, *Précis du cours d'économie politique* (Paris, 1878), p. 391.
2. Claude Tillier, *Mon oncle Benjamin* (Paris, 1881), p. 78. See also Louis Legrand, *Le Mariage et les moeurs en France* (Paris, 1879), p. 159 where the author cites the line from a poem by E. Angier in which a bourgeois says to his wife, "Nous pouvons nous donner le luxe d'un enfant."

3. Emile Faguet, . . . *et l'horreur des responsabilitiés* (Paris, 1911), pp. 134–145. See also Legrand, *Mariage*, p. 154.

4. Paul Bureau, "La propagande anticonceptionelle," *Revue pénitentiare et le droit pénal* 37 (1913), 720.

5. Cited in Pierre Deffontanes, *Les Hommes et leurs travaux dans les pays de la moyenne Garonne* (Lille, 1932), p. 103. See also Emmanuel Labat, *En Gascogne* (Agen, 1911), pp. 13–14.

6. Henri Baudrillart, *La Normandie, passé et present* (Paris, 1880), pp. 131, 136.

7. Georges Rocal, *Les Vieilles Coutumes dévotieuses et magiques du Perigord* (Toulouse, 1922), pp. 43–44; Jean Drouillet, *Folklore du Nivernais et du Morvan* (Charité sur Loire, 1959), p. 63; Dr. Boismoreau, *Coutumes médicales et superstitions populaires du bocage vendéen* (Paris, 1911), pp. 44–45.

8. Frederick Marshall, *Population and Trade in France in 1861—1862* (London, 1862), p. 34.

9. Jacques Bertillon, *La Dépopulation de la France* (Paris, 1911), pp. 107–109; Dr. Rommel, *Au pays de la revanche* (Geneva, 1886), p. 227. See also Marc Leproux, *Du berceau à la tombe* (Paris, 1959), pp. 7–8; Lucien Gachon, *L'Auvergne et le Velay* (Paris, 1948), pp. 316–317, and for a demographic analysis of regional variations Etienne van de Walle, *The Female Population of France in the Nineteenth Century* (Princeton, 1974).

10. *Bulletin de la société d'anthropologie de Paris* 7 (1896), 215 and see also the *Malthusian*, (December 1896), p. 93.

11. Maxime Leroy, *La Coutume Ouvrière* (Paris, 1913), 2:270. For general surveys of syndicalism see Peter N. Stearns, *Revolutionary Syndicalism and French Labor* (New Brunswick, N.J., 1971) and F.F. Ridley, *Revolutionary Syndicalism in France* (Cambridge, 1970).

12. Jean Maitron, *Histoire du mouvement anarchiste en France, 1880–1914* (Paris, 1955), pp. 249–311.

13. See Leroy, *Coutume*, 2:267–270; Christine Gras, *Alfred Rosmer 1877–1964* (Paris, 1970), pp. 38–39; Charles Desplanques, *La Voix du peuple*, (7 April 1910), p. 3; Louis Grandidier's assertion "the proletarians are tired of being proletarians, that is to say, makers of children" in *Voix du peuple*, (4 December 1910); p. 1; and on Franchet see *Génération consciente* (1 February 1909), p. 1.

14. On Verliac see Francis Ronsin, "La classe ouvrière et le néo-malthusianisme; l'exemple français avant 1914," *Mouvement social* 106 (1979), 85–117; and *Génération consciente* (September 1910).

15. See *Humanité* especially for the years 1908 to 1910.

16. On Roubaix see Bureau, "Propagande," pp. 714–715; on Fougères see Bernard Legendre, "La Vie d'un prolétariat: les ouvriers de Fougères au début du 20ᵉ siècle,"*Le Mouvement sociale* 98 (1977), 3–43 and *Génération consciente* (15 May 1908), p. 1; on Tourcoing see Bertillon, *Dépopulation*, p. 241; and on activists see *Régénération* (November 1903), p. 221; (January 1906), p. 146; *Génération consciente* (15 July 1908), (1 May 1909).

17. Bertillon, *Dépopulation*, pp. 219–222; René Béranger, "La Propagande néo-malthusienne," *La Réforme sociale* (1 August 1908), pp. 162—164. Bureau also noted a commercial house calling itself "Oeuvre maternelle médicale" which produced a journal entitled *Maternité* and sent birth control catalogues to new mothers. See Bureau, "Propagande," p. 723.

18. *Père Peinard*, (20—27 August 1893), p. 4.

19. Jehan Rictus, *Le Coeur populaire* (Paris, n.d.), p. 205.

20. Cited by R.H. Guerrand, *La Libre Maternité 1896–1969* (Paris, 1971), p. 55. Alphonse Gallais' "Remède à la misère" presented much the same message as Clement.
21. Cited by Andrè Armengaud, *Les Français et Malthus* (Paris, 1975), p. 57. According to Charles Deplanques the bourgeois dissuaded his wife from having children with the phrase, "Fi donc, ma chère, c'est bon pour les ouvriers." *La Voix du peuple* (7 April 1910), p. 3.
22. Maurice Beaufreton, *Le Logement populaire à Paris* (Paris, 1898), p. 301.
23. Dr. Octave du Mesnil and Dr. Charles Mangenot, *Etude hygiénique et d'économie sociale* (Paris, 1899), p. 89.
24. du Mesnil, *Étude*, pp. 89–90.
25. René Martial, *Hygiène individuelle du travailleur* (Paris, 1907), p. 214.
26. du Mesnil, *Étude*, p. 89.
27. Madeleine Vernet, "Toujours sur l'avortement," *Les Temps nouveaux* (1 April 1911), p. 1. On the expense of birth control appliances which would limit their use in workers' homes, see Pierre Pierrard, *La Vie ouvrière à Lille sous le second empire* (Paris, 1965), p. 124.
28. *Régénération* (June 1904), p. 280.
29. Cited in Standish Meacham, *A Life Apart: The English Working Class 1890–1914* (London, 1977), p. 70.
30. *Régénération* (July 1902), p. 90. In contrast, see the argument that the working-class wife enjoyed greater power in the family than the middle-class wife in Jeanne Deflou, *Le Sexualisme: critique de la prépondérance et de la mentalité du sexe forte* (Paris, 1906), pp. 147–148.
31. Martial, *Hygiène*, p. 216.
32. *La Guerre sociale* (1 July 1914), p. 2; (24 June 1914), p. 2; (8 July 1914), p. 2; (22 July 1914), p. 2 and for an early appreciation of Hervé see *Génération consciente* (May 1910).
33. *La Guerre sociale* (17 June 1914), p. 1; (29 July 1914), p. 4 and see also (15 July 1914), p. 4 and (22 July 1914), p. 3.
34. Bureau, "Propagande," p. 716.
35. Bertillon, *Dépopulation*, p. 216.
36. Fernand Boverat, *Patriotisme et paternité* (Paris, 1913), pp. 322–335.
37. *Année sociale internationale* 4 (1913–1914) 110–111.
38. Béranger, "Propagande," p. 170. See also the assertion of Etienne Lamy, "The propaganda in favor of free and infertile unions was aimed with the greatest intensity at women workers. It is in the industrial cities that the campaign for sterility has caused the greatest damage." "La flamme qui ne doit s'éteindre," *Revue des deux mondes* 42 (1917), 539.

CHAPTER NINE

1. E.A. Wrigley, "Family Limitation in Pre-industrial England," *Economic History Review* 19 (1966), 105, n. 3.
2. Norman B. Ryder, "The Character of Modern Fertility," *The Annals of the American Academy of Political and Social Science* 359 (1967), 29.
3. Henri Estienne, *L'Introduction au traité de la conformité des merveilles anciennes avec les modernes* (Paris, 1566), p. 256.

4. Cited in Jules Royer, *Études médicales sur l'ancienne Rome* (Paris, 1859), p. 195.

5. Charles de Montesquieu, *De l'esprit des loix* (Paris, 1748), chapt. 23, pp. 16, 17; J.J. Rousseau, *Émile ou l'éducation: Oeuvres complètes* (Paris, 1958), 3:25; Marquis de Sade, *La Philosophie dans la boudoir* (Londres, 1795), 1:66–67.

6. Moheau [A.J.B.R. Auget de Montyon?], *Recherches et considérations sur la population de la France* (Paris, 1773), 2:100. See also Philippe Hecquet, *La Médecine, la chirurgie et la pharmacie des pauvres* (Paris, 1839), p. 215.

7. Referring to the upsurge of eighteenth-century legislation on abortion, Suzanne Dreyer-Roos states, "Toutes ces mesures visaient principalement les 'personnes engrossées hors les liens du mariage' dont les agissements se trouvaient suspects." *La Population strasbourgeoise sous l'ancien régime* (Paris, 1969), p. 192. See also Olwen Hufton, *The Poor of Eighteenth Century France* (Oxford, 1974), p. 331. Prostitutes were a special class that was always credited with a knowledge of abortive techniques; see Mathurin Régnier, *Les Satyrs: oeuvres complètes* (Paris, 1958), pp. 160–161; A.J.B. Parent-Duchatelet, *De la prostitution dans la ville de Paris* (Paris, 1836), passim; Alphonse Esquiros, *Les Vierges folles* (Paris, 1842), p. 101.

8. Louis Chevalier, *Classes laborieuses et classes dangereuses à Paris pendant la première moitié du XIXe siècle* (Paris, 1958), p. 332; Jean Vidalenc, *La Société français de 1815 à 1848* (Paris, 1969–1973), 2:396–406.

9. Gérando, *Le Visiteur du pauvre* (Paris, 1820), pp. 86–87.

10. Adolphe Blanqui, *Cours d'économie industrielle* (Paris, 1838), 1:147; C.T. Duchâtel, *La Charité* (Paris, 1829); J.F. Terme and M. Monfalcon, *Histoire des enfants trouvés* (Paris, 1840); Bernard-Benoit Remacle, *Rapport concernant les infanticides* (Paris, 1845).

11. Alphonse Esquiros, *Paris, ou les sciences, les institutions, et les moeurs au XIXe siècle* (Paris, 1847), 2:355. See also Alphonse Devergie, *Annales d'hygiène publique*, IV (1830), 4:193–205; Ernest Legouvé, *Histoire morale des femmes* (Paris, 1849), p. 328.

12. Vidal, *De la répartition des richesses* (Paris, 1846), p. 285. See also P. Pradier-Fodéré, *Précis de droit politique et d'économie sociale* (Paris, 1859), p. 366.

13. Emile de Girardin, *La Liberté dans le mariage* (Paris, 1854); Louis Viallet, *Rapport au préfet et au conseil général de l'Aveyron sur les institutions charitables* (Espallion, 1860); Ambroise Tardieu, *Étude médico-légale sur l'infanticide* (Paris, 1868).

14. M. Chatagnier, *De l'infanticide* (Paris, 1855), p. 10.

15. *Le Contribuable* (December 1866) cited in Dr. F. Brochard, *La Vérité sur les enfants trouvés* (Paris, 1876); p. 102. See also Dr. P. Brouardel, *L'Infanticide* (Paris, 1897).

16. Brochard, *La Vérité*, p. 18.

17. Cited in Brochard, *La Vérité*, p. 98.

18. Brochard, *La Vérité*, pp. 98–99. See also Dr. F. Brochard, *Des Causes de la dépopulation en France et les moyens d'y remédier* (Lyon, 1873), p. 17.

19. Albert Dupoux, *Sur les pas de Monsieur Vincent: trois cents ans d'histoire parisienne de l'enfance abandonnée* (Paris, 1958), pp. 187–201.

20. It was noteworthy that Charles Knowlton's birth control tract, *Fruits of Philosophy*, was entitled *Plus d'avortements!* in its French translation. Such condemnations of abortion were often made only for tactical reasons; some French neo-Malthusians would defend the practice in the first decade of the twentieth century. See footnotes 72 and 80.

21. Paul Leroy-Beaulieu, *La question de la dépopulation* (Paris, 1913), p. 298.

22. Paul Bureau, "La Propagande anticonceptionnelle," *Revue pénitentiare et de droit pénal* 37 (1913), p. 714. On class differences see also Henri Baudrillart, *La Normandie, passé et present* (Paris, 1880), p. 127.

23. Cited in Charles Gide, "Le Dépeuplement de la France," *La Revue hebdomadaire* 19 (8 May 1909), 143.

24. On the medical history of abortion in France see François Mauriceau, *Traité des maladies des femmes et de celles qui sont accouchées* (Paris, 1712), p. 338; F.E. Fodéré, *Traité de médecine légale* (Paris, 1813) 2:64−68; 4:381ff.; Alph. Devergie, "Avortement," *Dictionnaire de médecine et de chirurgie pratique* (Paris, 1829), pp. 674−678; G.N. Notte, *Considérations médico-légales sur les causes de l'avortement prétendu criminel* (Aix, 1833); Paul Dubois, "De l'avortement provoqué dans les cas de rétrécissement du basin," *Gazette médicale* 9(4 March 1843), pp. 135−139; C.C. Brillaud-Laujardière, *De l'avortement provoqué* (Paris, 1862); Emile Garimond, *Traité théorique et pratique de l'avortement* (Paris, 1901).

25. M. Lenoir, "Observations d'avortement provoqué pour la troisième fois avec succès, suivie de quelques réflexions relatives à cette operation," *Bulletin de l'Académie de médecine* 17 (10 February 1852), 364−390, (2 March 1852), 467−472, (9 March 1852), 493−503.

26. J.L. Baudelocque, *Two Memoirs on the Caesarian Operation,* trans. John Hull (Manchester, 1801), pp. 10−11. See also J.L. Baudelocque, "Recherches sur l'opération césarienne," *Recueil périoḍique de la société de médecine de Paris* 5 (1797), 1−89; J. Capuron, *La Médecine légale relative à l'art des accouchements* (Paris, 1821), p. 291 and *Cours théorique et pratique d'accouchements* (Paris, 1828), pp. 497, 551.

27. On the church and abortion, see Archbishop Gousset, *Théologie morale à l'usage des curés et des confesseurs* (Paris, 1844); P.J.C. Debreyne, *Essai sur la théologie morale considerée dans ses rapports avec la physiognomie et la médecine,* 5th ed. (Paris, 1868), p. 200; Le Baron F. Dunot de Saint Maclou, *Du Foeticide médical* (Caen, 1860) and also *Lettre à M. le docteur Lemenant des Chesnais* (Caen, 1861); Ph. Passot, "Études et observations obstétricales," *Gazette médicale de Lyon* (1853); pp. 25−28; Edgar de Vesine Larue, *Essai sur l'avortement* (Paris, 1866); Adolphe Pinard, *Du foeticide* (Paris, 1901).

28. *Le Voltaire* (7 November 1890), p. 1. On doctors and morality, see also Abbé Camille Ract, *Natalité* (Paris, 1901), p. 217.

29. Ambroise Tardieu, *Étude médico-légale sur l'avortement,* 5th ed. (Paris, 1898), p. 5.

30. For examples of advertisements, see Jacques Bertillon, *La Dépopulation de la France* (Paris, 1911), pp. 243−244; Dr. Madeleine Pelletier, *Le Droit d'avortement* (Paris, 1913), p. 8.

31. Félix Allemane, *L'Avortement criminel* (Carcassonne, 1911), p. 121; Rouyer, *Études médicales,* p. 78.

32. Gustave Drouineau, *Rapport sur l'influence des avortements criminels sur la dépopulation et les mesures à prendre* (Melun, 1908), p. 11.

33. E. Verrier, "L'avortement criminel chez les anciens les modernes," *La Revue scientifique de la France et de l'étranger* 7 (1884); 793.

34. Pelletier, *Le Droit,* p. 9.

35. M. Barthélemy, "Répression de l'avortement criminel," *Revue pénitentiare et de droit pénal* 41 (1917), 104−113.

36. In 1913 the 200 women at the hôpital Boucicault who admitted to having had an abortion declared that the operation had been carried out in 39 cases by midwives, in 27 by doctors or medical students, in 3 by pharmacists, in 12 by herbalists, in 24 by nurses, in 21 by the women themselves, in 74 by nonmedical personnel. Dr. G. Lepage, "A propos des avortements criminels à Paris," *La Revue philanthropique* 38

(1917), 493. For hostile literary presentations of the abortionist, see Alexandre Dumas fils, *La Femme de Claude* (Paris, 1873), p. 40; Alexandre Boutique, *Les Malthusiennes* (Paris, 1894), p. 105; Emile Zola, *Fécondité* (Paris, 1890). For sympathetic portrayals, see footnote 80.

37. For accounts of doctors accused of abortion, see M. Halmagrand, *Considérations médico-légales sur l'avortement* (Paris, 1844); Dr. Charles Vibert, "L'Affaire du docteur Lafitte," *Annales d'hygiène publique et de médecine légale* 32 (1894), 349–362.

38. Henri Bérenger, *Les Prolétaires intellectuelles en France* (Paris, 1901), P. 8. See also Armand Hayem, *Le Mariage* (Paris, 1872), p. 158.

39. Tardieu, *Étude médico-légale*, passim. Savine, a herb used by midwives to induce labor, enjoyed the greatest reputation as an abortifacient. See E. Ferdut, *De l'avortement au point de vue médical, obstétrical, médico-légal, légal et théologique* (Paris, 1865), pp. 81–88; A. Boissard and G. Barbezieux, *Mères et nourrisons* (Paris, 1892), p. 33; Max Caisson, "Le Four et l'araignée," *Ethnologie française* 6 (1976), 374–375. On ergot, see Christine Poitou, "Ergotisme, ergot de seigle et épidémies en Sologne au 18ᵉ siècle," *Revue d'histoire moderne et contemporaine* 23 (1976), 365—366. On rue see Paul Sebillot, *Le Folk-lore de France* (Paris, 1968), 3:501.

40. M.B. Lavigne, *Histoire de Blagnac* (Toulouse, 1875), p. 373.

41. Chatagnier, *De L'infanticide*, p. 259. See also Max. Simon, *Déontologie médicale ou des devoirs et des droits des médecins* (Paris, 1845), pp. 478–479.

42. Cited in A. Hamon, *La France sociale et politique: 1891* (Paris, 1892), p. 629.

43. Boismoreau, *Coutumes médicales*, p. 44.

44. On urban working-class women and abortion, see C. Granier, *La Femme criminelle* (1906), pp. 83ff.; Bureau, "La Propagande," p. 714; Ernest Bertrand, "Essai sur la moralité des classes ouvrières dans leur vie privée," *Journal de la société de statistique de Paris* (April 1873) pp. 86ff.; Emile Brousse, *Débats parlementaires: Chambre des députés* (1891), p. 231; Mme. Paul de Schlumberger, *Aux jeunes ouvrières* (Paris, 1911), p. 22.

45. Chatagnier, *De l'infanticide*, pp. 258–259.

46. Hubert Legrand, "Deux Mots sur les avortements criminels," *Revue professionnelle des sages-femmes* (February 1911), p. 26.

47. Granier, *La Femme criminelle*, p. 101

48. Marcelle Bouteillier, *Médecine populaire d'hier et d'aujourd'hui* (Paris, 1966), p. 306.

49. Droineau, *Rapport*, p. 8.

50. Pelletier, *Le Droit*, p. 10.

51. G.M. Savarit, "Le dépeuplement de la France," *La Revue hebdomadaire* (1909), p. 258.

52. Burlureux, "Le dépeuplement de la France," *La revue hebdomadaire* (1909), p. 430.

53. Ibid., p. 431. For similar reports of "cynicism," see T. Gallard, *De l'avortement au point de vue médico-légale* (Paris, 1878), p. 15. On the problem of professional secrecy and abortion, see Dr. P. Brouardel, *Le Secret médical* (Paris, 1887), pp. 162–163; C. Colson, "La Tache de demain — la population," *Revue des deux mondes* 26 (15 April 1915), 873.

54. Dr. P.A. Lop, *Conférence sur le secret professionnel et l'avortement criminel* (Paris, 1905), p. 6.

55. Barthélemy, "Répression de l'avortement," p. 104.

56. A. Lacassagne, *Précis de la médecine légale* (Paris, 1906), p. 823.

57. In Ferri-Pisani's novel *Stérilité!* (Paris, 1906), p. 21, a midwife abortionist informs her patient that doctors can easily induce a miscarriage: "C'est aussi simple que bonjour."

An American physician visiting Paris reported seeing abortive instruments openly sold. Frederick Griffith, "Instruments for the Production of Abortion Sold in the Market Places of Paris," *Medical Record* (January 30, 1904), pp. 171–172.

58. Dr. Munaret, *Du médecin des villes et du médecin de campagne* (Paris, 1840), p. 427. See also Fodéré, *Traité*, 4:388.

59. In 1908 the Congrès d'obstétrique heard reports that up to one-third of all conceptions were being aborted, but in the same year only twenty-five abortionists were tried. See Joseph Reinach, *Débats parlementaires: Chambre des députés* (1909), p. 3610. On the figures available see Jacques Léauté, *Recherches sur l'infanticide, Annales de la faculté de droit et des sciences politiques et économiques de Strasbourg*, Cahier 17 (Paris, 1968).

60. Robert Michels, *Sexual Ethics* (London, 1914), p. 261.

61. Brochard, *La Vérité*, pp. 99–100.

62. Tardieu, *Étude médico-légale*, passim.

63. On trials see A. Hamon, *La France*, pp. 629–630 and *La France: 1890* (Paris, 1890), 2:295.

64. *La Chronique médicale* (15 February 1909), p. 120.

65. For the figures on abortion see Dr. Balthazard and Eugène Prévost, *Une Plaie sociale (les avortements criminels)*, (Paris, 1912), p. 39; Lacassagne, *Précis*, p. 825; S. du Moriez, *L'Avortement* (Paris, 1912), pp. 25–26; Barthélemy, "Répression de l'avortement," p. 6; Leroy-Beaulieu, *La Question*, p. 329; Robert Talmy, *Histoire du mouvement familiale en France (1896–1939)* (Paris, 1962), 1:129–130.

66. See Dr. Courtault, *Pourquoi l'avortement précoce doit être médicalement libre* (Paris, 1909), p. 3.

67. Early in the century there had been a call in Dezeimeris and Desormeaux, "Avortement," *Dictionnaire de médecine* (1833), 4:475 for a reform of the harsh law of 1810 if only to make it easier to secure the convictions of abortionists.

68. E. Adolph Spiral, *Essai d'une Etude sur l'avortement* (Paris, 1882), p. 13.

69. Auguste Forel, *La Question sexuelle exposées aux adultes cultivés*, 3rd ed. (Paris, 1911) pp. 468, 506–507.

70. Dr. Léon Dumas, *L'Interdiction de la recherche de la paternité et l'avortement provoqué criminellement* (Nimes, 1903). See also Gustave Rivet, *La Recherche de la paternité* (1890), p. 139; Daniel Riche, *Les Drames du mariage: L'article 340* (Paris, n.d.).

71. Dr. Antoine Wylm, *La Morale Sexuelle* (Paris, 1907), pp. 206–209.

72. For the opinions of Alfred Naquet, the tireless advocate of divorce and similar social reforms, see the referendum held on the subject by *La Chronique médicale* (15 February 1909), pp. 97–132 and (15 April 1909), pp. 255–269. Of the doctors who replied, 111 were in favor of retention of the existing law, 7 for its modification, and 5 for its abrogation. See also M. Gand, "Un Referendum sur l'avortement," *Revue pénitenciare et de droit penal* 33 (1909), p. 1284; G. Hardy, *La Loi de Malthus* (Paris, 1909), p. 35; Dr. Klotz-Forest, *De l'avortement: est-ce un crime?* (Paris, 1919).

73. Cited in Bernard Lecache, *Séverine* (Paris, 1930), pp. 88–89. For the outburst of radical sympathy expressed for the women inculpated in the trial of the abortionist known as "La mort aux gosses," see *Gil blas illustré* (29 November 1891), pp. 1–2; see also the cartoon "L'avortée," by A. Willette in *Le Courrier français* (22 November 1891), p. 1 and Charles Léandre's cartoon "La faiseuse d'anges," in Gustave Kahn, *La Femme dans la caricature française* (Paris, 1912), p. 24. For the Banks' thesis see J.A. and O. Banks, *Feminism and Family Planning* (New York, 1964).

74. Lux, "Un crime que l'on ne punit plus," *Revue bleue* 9 (23 May 1909), 671—672; see also Edmond Deschaumes, *La Banqueroute de l'amour* (Paris, 1896), pp. 49–50.

75. Dr. E. Toulouse, *Les Conflits intersexuels et sociaux* (Paris, 1904), p. 322.

76. Cited in Allemane, *L'Avortement*, p. 127.

77. Courtault, *L'avortement précoce*, passim. There is no space to discuss the enormous antiabortion, pronatalist literature of the period but see Georges Blet, *L'Avortement. Est-ce un crime? Sa répression est-elle légitime?* (Macon, 1911); P.A. Vuillermet, *Le Suicide d'une race* (Paris, 1911); *Revue de l'alliance nationale pour l'accroisement de la population française* (Paris, 1922); Victoria Giraud, *Le Suicide de la France* (Paris, 1923).

78. Pelletier, *Le Droit*, p. 7.

79. Ibid., p. 7. See also Dr. J. Darricarrère, *Droit à l'avortement* (Paris, 1906). The German socialist leader August Bebel had noted earlier in the century that in France the conscientious, not just the frivolous, women had recourse to abortion. August Bebel, *Woman. Her Position in the Past, Present, and Future* (London, 1893), pp. 62–63.

80. Daniel Riche, *Stérile* (Paris, n.d.) cited in the *Malthusian* (October 1899), p. 76. For other defenses of abortion and abortionists in literature see Eugène Brieux, *Maternity*, trans. Mrs. George Bernard Shaw (London, 1907); Ferri-Pisani, *Stérilité* (Paris, 1906); Michel Corday, *Sésame, ou la maternité consentie* (Paris, 1903); André Couvreur, *La Famille: la graine* (Paris, 1902).

81. Edward Shorter, "Female Emancipation, Birth Control, and Fertility in European History," *American Historical Review* 88 (1973), 629; Joan W. Scott and Louise Tilly, "Women's Work and the Family in Nineteenth Century Europe," in Charles E. Rosenberg, ed., *The Family in History* (Philadelphia, 1975), p. 168.

82. See George D. Sussman, "The Wet-nursing Business in Nineteenth-Century France," *French Historical Studies* 9 (1975), 304–328.

83. Lawrence Wylie, *Village in the Vaucluse* (New York, 1961), pp. 335–336; Stanley Hoffman et al. *In Search of France* (New York, 1963), passim. On the concept of "domestic feminism" see Daniel S. Smith, "Family Limitation, Sexual Control, and Domestic Feminism in Victorian America," in M. Hartman and L.W. Banner, eds., *Clio's Consciousness Raised* (New York, 1974).

CHAPTER TEN

1. Emma Goldman, *Living My Life* (New York, 1931), pp. 272–273. In the account of the August 4–6, 1900, meeting *Régénération* described Goldman as a San Francisco midwife.

2. Père Féline, *Catéchisme des gens mariés* (Caen, 1782), pp. 41–42; on Bouvier, see chapter two above.

3. G. Vacher de Lapouge, *Les Sélections sociales* (Paris, 1896), p. 361. Another enemy of feminism, Charles Turgeon, suggested that women's emancipation and the decline of fertility were related physiologically; the educated woman used up her "force nerveuse" and consequently became sterile. See Turgeon, *Le Féminisme français* (Paris, 1907), 1:315.

4. Paul Leroy-Beaulieu, *Traité théorique et pratique d'économie politique* (Paris, 1896), 4:623–628.

5. Georges Rossignol, *Un Pays de célibataires et de fils unique* (Paris, 1913), p. 111.

6. Abbé Camille Ract, *Natalité* (Paris, 1901), pp. 163ff.

7. Jacques Lux, "Un Crime que l'on ne punit plus," *Revue bleu* 9 (23 May 1908), pp. 671–672; *Journal officiel. Débats parlementaires. Chambre de députés* (25 November 1909), p. 2931.

8. Etienne Lamy, "La Flamme qui ne doit pas s'éteindre," *Revue des deux mondes* 42 (1917), 265.

9. Dr. J.A. Doléris and Jean Bouscatel, *Néo-malthusianisme: maternité et féminisme: éducation sexuelle* (Paris, 1918), p. 23.

10. Stanley Hoffman et al., *In Search of France* (New York, 1964).

11. John and Olive Banks, *Feminism and Family Planning* (New York, 1964).

12. Claire Moses, "The Evolution of Feminist Thought in France, 1829–1889," unpublished Ph.D. dissertation (George Washington University, 1978).

13. Désirée Gay, *Opinion* (21 August 1848) cited in Moses, "Feminist Thought," p. 298. Désirée Veret, a friend of Suzanne Voilquin, went to Britain where she was involved with the Owenites and then returned to Paris where she married the Fourierist Leopold Gay.

14. On the feminism of the first half of the nineteenth century, see Marguerite Thibert, *Le Féminisme dans le socialisme française de 1830 à 1850* (Paris, 1926); Léon Absenour, *Le Féminisme sous le régne de Louis-Philippe* (Paris, 1913); S. Joan Moon, "The Saint-Simonian Association of Working-Class Women, 1830–1850," *Proceedings of the Fifth Annual Meeting of the Western Association for French History, 1977* (Santa Barbara, 1978), pp. 274–281.

15. Suzanne Voilquin in Preface to Claire Démar, *Ma Loi d'avenir* (Paris, 1834) in Valentin Pelousse, ed., *Claire Démar: Textes sur l'affranchissement des femmes, 1832–1833* (Paris, 1976), p. 164. Démar committed suicide with her lover Perret Desessarts in August 1833; her work appeared posthumously the following year.

16. Voilquin, *Ma Loi*, p. 165.

17. Gay, *Voix* (19 April 1848) cited in Moses, "Feminist Thought," p. 163.

18. Edith Thomas, *Pauline Roland: socialisme et féminisme au 19ᵉ siècle* (Paris, 1956), pp. 64–65.

19. Valentin, *Démar*, pp. 93–94.

20. Flora Tristan, *Promenades dans Londres* (Paris, 1840), p. 313.

21. On women and work, see Marilyn J. Boxer, "Foyer or Factory: Working-Class Women in Nineteenth-Century France," *Proceedings of the Second Annual Meeting of the Western Association for French History, 1974* (Santa Barbara, 1975); Joan W. Scott and Louise Tilly, *Women, Work and the Family* (New York, 1978).

22. Theodore Zeldin, *France, 1848—1945* (London, 1973), 2:351; 2:973.

23. André Leo [Leodile de Champceix], *La Femme et les moeurs* (Paris, 1860), pp. 49–53, 104. For attacks on Michelet, see also Adèle Esquiros, *L'Amour* (Paris, 1860).

24. Jenny P. d'Hericourt, *La Femme affranchie* (Paris, 1860), 1:91–126. In response to the assertions of Comte and Proudhon that political freedoms for women would be translated into sexual libertinism, d'Hericourt replied, "To emancipate the woman is not to recognize her right of using and abusing love."

25. Juliette Lamber [Juliette Adam], *Idées anti-proudhoniennes sur l'amour, la femme et le mariage* (Paris, 1861), p. 77. On the woman's right to work, see also Mlle. J.V. Daubie, *La Femme pauvre au 19ᵉ siècle* (Paris, 1866), pp. 341–345.

26. Paul Robin cited by Gabriel Giroud, *Paul Robin* (Paris, 1937), p. 214.

27. *Régénération* (June 1904), p. 124.

28. See chapter eight.

29. *Malthusian* (March 1897), p. 18.

30. On Huot, see the introduction by Rachilde to Huot's book of poems — many addressed to "les anges de foyer," her cats — *Le Missel de Notre Dame des solitudes* (Paris, 1908).

31. There is no adequate study of the antivivisection movement in France but for Anglo-Saxon countries, see John Vyvyan, *In Pity and in Anger: A Study of the Use of Animals in Science* (New York, 1969); R.D. French, *Antivivisection and Medical Science in Victorian Society* (Princeton, 1975).

32. For an account of Huot's lecture, see *L'Encylopédie contemporaine illustré* (9 October 1892), p. 280; *Le Temps* (4 October 1892), p. 1.

33. In a letter published in *Génération consciente* (November 1909) Huot gave her recollections of the 1892 speech and added the ethnocentric comment that repeated pregnancies might be tolerated by orientals but not by occidentals.

34. See *La Fronde* (28 May 1892), p. 2; (6 April 1903), p. 2; (24 March 1903), p. 1; (24 January 1903), p. 1.

35. On *Régénération's* welcome given to the support by Petit, see the columns of August 1904. See also the defense of the woman's right to decide on the timing of maternity given by Maria Martin, editor of *Journal des femmes* (August–September 1903).

36. *Action* in fact provided issues of Drysdale's *Eléments* as prizes for its readers.

37. On Roussel, see her articles collected in *Quelque lances rompues pour nos libertés* (Paris, 1910).

38. Roussel's feminist appeal of 1903 was reprinted by syndicalist papers such as *Le Relieur, Le Combat de Levallois-Clichy*, and *L'Ouvrier métallurgiste*.

39. See Dr. Madeleine Pelletier, *Le droit à l'avortement* (Paris, 1913) and *L'Amour et la maternité* (Paris, n.d.)

40. See also Marilyn J. Boxer, "Socialism Faces Feminism: The Failure of a Synthesis in France, 1879–1914," in Boxer and Jean H. Quataert, *Socialist Women: European Socialist Feminism in the Nineteenth and Twentieth Centuries* (New York, 1978), pp. 75–111.

41. See Moses, "French Feminism," passim.

42. Mme. Abaddie d'Arrast, the president of the Conseil national des femmes, was frequently attacked by Robin and his followers for her conservatism.

43. Auclert, *Les Femmes au gouvernail* (Paris, 1923), p. 309. Mme. Schlumberger similarly attacked the birth control movement in the *International Women's Suffrage News*. See the *Malthusian* (September 1917).

44. See Boxer and Quataert, *Socialism*, pp. 75–111; Charles Sowerine, "The Organization of French Socialist Women, 1880–1914; A European Perspective for Women's Movements," *Historical Reflections* 3 (1976), 3–24 and his "Le groupe féministe socialiste, 1892–1902," *le Mouvement social* 90 (1975), 87–120.

45. On Austria see Boxer and Quataert, *Socialism*, pp. 241–243; on Germany, Jean H. Quataert, *Reluctant Feminists in German Social Democracy, 1885–1917* (Princeton, 1979), pp. 95–99; Richard J. Evans, *The Feminist Movement in Germany, 1894–1933* (London, 1976).

46. Aline Valette and M. Bonnier, *Socialisme et sexualisme* (Paris, 1893).

47. Paul Robin, *Libre Amour, libre maternité* (Paris, 1900), p. 2. Leopold Lacour spoke at the same conference; see his *Humanisme intégral* (Paris, 1897), pp. 284ff.in which birth control is defended.

48. *Régénération* (January 1907), (March 1907), (August 1905). Manuel Devaldès asserted in *Régénération* (August 1908) that all the "feministes pures" were bourgeois.

49. See *La Femme affranchie*, (June, August 1905); (May 1908).

50. On the diffusion of birth control, see Léon Legavre, *La Femme dans la société* (Paris, 1907), pp. 441ff.

51. Margaret Sanger, *An Autobiography* (New York, 1938), p. 104. The French influence on the early stages of the American birth control movement can be gauged by the references to M. Marestan, Victor Méric, and Louise Michel in Sanger's *Woman Rebel* (1914).

CHAPTER ELEVEN

1. Colin Dyer, *Population and Society in Twentieth Century France* (London, 1978), p. 56.

2. Dr. Rommel, *Au pays de la revanche* (Geneva, 1886), p. 227; see also Claude Digeon, *La Crise allemande de la pensée française, 1870—1914* (Paris, 1959).

3. Jean Boillot, *Le Pays de la revanche et le pays des milliards: réponse au Dr. Rommel* (Neuchâtel, 1886), p. 205.

4. Georges Rossignol, *Un Pays de célibataires et de fils unique* (Paris, 1913), p. 322.

5. Fernand Boverat, *Patriotisme et paternité* (Paris, 1913), p. 322.

6. Gustave Le Bon, *Les Lois physiologiques de l'évolution des peuples* (Paris, 1894), pp. 160—164; G. Vacher de Lapouge, *Les Sélections sociales* (Paris, 1896), pp. 188—194.

7. Dr. Alexandre Picon, *Aperçu sur les principales causes de la dépopulation* (Paris, 1888), pp. 6—9; Dr. E. Maurel, *De la dépopulation de la France* (Paris, 1896), p. 233; Raoul de Félice, *Les Naissances en France* (Paris, 1910), pp. 101—127.

8. For attacks on doctors see Etienne Lamy, "La flamme qui ne doit pas s'éteindre," *Revue des deux mondes* 42 (1917), 530; D.M. Couturier, *Demain: la dépopulation de la France: craintes et espérances* (1901), p. 59; Camille Ract, *Natalité* (Paris, 1901), p. 217. For attacks on the church see Lapouge, *Sélections*, p. 191; Rossignol, *Un Pays*, p. 302.

9. Georges Deherme, *Croître ou disparaître* (Paris, 1910), pp. 75—77.

10. On Frederic Passy see *Malthusian* (March 1897), p. 17.

11. *Bulletin de la société d'anthropologie de Paris* 7 (1896), 138—140.

12. For the views of loyal Malthusians such as Lavergne, Molinari, and Caudrelier see J.J. Spengler, *France Faces Depopulation* (Durham, N.C., 1938), p. 141.

13. Le Play's main works were *La Réforme sociale en France* (Paris, 1866) and *Les ouvriers européens* (Paris, 1879). See also Spengler, *France*, p. 146 and Michael Z. Brooke, *Le Play: Engineer and Social Scientist* (London, 1970).

14. Dumont's main works were *Dépopulation et civilisation* (Paris, 1890) and *Natalité et démocratie* (Paris, 1898). See also Spengler, *France*, p. 156; Theodore Zeldin, *France, 1848—1945* (Oxford, 1976), 2:964; Camille Rabaud, *Le Péril national ou la dépopulation de la France* (Paris, 1891).

15. *Bulletin de la société d'anthroplogie de Paris* 7 (1896), 142.

16. Emile Durkheim, *Le Suicide* (Paris, 1897), pp. 208—214.

17. Paul Leroy-Beaulieu, *Traité théorique et pratique d'économie politique* (Paris, 1896) 4:518; and see also his *La Question de la population* (Paris, 1913).

18. Leroy-Beaulieu, *Traité*, p. 518.

19. See Ernest Cadet, *Le Mariage en France* (Paris, 1870), pp. 48—52; A. de Fouillée, "Le Dépeuplement de la France," *Revue hebdomadaire* (1909), p. 17; Charles Lyon-Caen, "Le Dépeuplement de la France et la législation civile," *Revue hebdomadaire* (1909), p. 560.

20. See the discussion of "recherche de paternité" in chapter ten above and also Lyon-Caen, "Le dépeuplement," p. 570; P. Cauwès, *Précis du cours d'économie*

politique (Paris, 1878), p. 405. On opposition to reform, see Lucien A. Cazals, *Les Grands criminals sociaux au 20ᵉ siècle* (Toulouse, 1903), p. 21; Edmond Deschaumes, *La Banqueroute de l'amour* (Paris, 1896).

21. Lyon-Caen, "Le Dépeuplement," p. 578.

22. See Edme Piot, *La Dépopulation* (Paris, 1902); Boverat, *Patriotisme* pp. 205–207; P. Cuzacq, *La Naissance, le mariage et le décès* (Paris, 1902) p. 35; Auguste Lainé, *De la dépopulation de la France* (Paris, 1891), p. 50. On opposition to such reforms see *Génération consciente* (15 September 1908) *Régénération* (January 1901), p. 3; Henri Dagan, *L'Oeuvre nouvelle*, (1903–1904), p. 80.

23. See René Martial, *Hygiène individuelle du travailleur* (Paris, 1907); Beaufreton, *Le Logement populaire à Paris* (Paris, 1898), p. 301; Boverat, *Patriotisme*, p. 205.

24. Paul Strauss, *Dépopulation et puériculture* (Paris, 1901); Henri de Rothschild, *Dépopulation et problème de la première enfance* (Paris, 1901). On the general concern for child care, see Luc Boltanski, *Prime Education et morale de classe* (Paris, 1969).

25. See Cuzacq, *La Naissance*, p. 40; Maurel, *De la dépopulation*, pp. 185–186; Jules Jung, *Des moyens actuellement proposées pour favoriser l'accroissement de la natalité en France* (Paris, 1903), pp. 56 ff; Gustave Rouanet, "La dépopulation de la France," *Revue socialiste* 10 (1889), 396.

26. On the general movement see André Armengaud, *Les Français et Malthus* (Paris, 1975). For the attacks of the neo-Malthusians on "les puritards," "les grippeminauds," who, in Nelly Roussel's estimation should have been prosecuted for "encouragement of bestiality," see *Régénération* (August 1900) p. 3; *Génération consciente*, (May 1909).

27. On Fallot see Marc Boegner, *La Vie et la pensée de T. Fallot* (Paris, 1914–1926), 2 vols.; on Bérenger, see R.H. Guerrand, *La Libre Maternité, 1896–1969* (Paris, 1971), pp. 55 ff.; Jeanne Humbert, *Eugène Humbert: la vie et l'oeuvre d'un néo-malthusien* (Paris, 1947), p. 85; René Béranger, "La propagande néo-Malthusienne," *La Réforme sociale* (1 August 1908), p. 161 ff. For attacks on the movement see *Malthusian*, (July 1900), p. 54; *Régénération* (July 1901), p. 6.

28. See the special undated flyer put out in the summer of 1897 by *Régénération* opposing the projected Béranger bill. See also Gide's contribution to the *Revue hebdomadaire* (May 1909), pp. 141–148 and on Gide's other activities, see Sanford Elwitt, "Social Reform and Social Order in Late Nineteenth Century France: the Musée social and Its Friends," *French Historical Studies* (1980), 11:431–451.

29. On Bureau, see the *Malthusian*, (April 1912), p. 321; and his contributions to "La propagande anticonceptionelle," *Revue pénitenciare et de droit pénal* 37 (1913), 713–749, 1169–1199; and *Année sociale internationale* 4 (1913–1914), 108–114; and his *L'Indiscipline des moeurs* (Paris, 1920).

30. J. Bertillon, *La Dépopulation de la France* (Paris, 1911), pp. 210–213; and see also *Malthusian* (October 1896), p. 73.

31. See *La Revue de l'Alliance* (1922). On Michelin paternalism, see Cicely Hamilton, *Modern France: As Seen by an Englishwoman* (London, 1933), pp. 19–25.

32. E. de Blic, *Nous les aurons. Mais après. . . ? Aux "Poilus" pour le lendemain de la victoire. Conférence donnée dans un cantonnement du front le 6 juillet 1916* (Paris, 1916), p. 23.

33. Blic, *Nous*, p. 33. For similar sentiments see Alfred Krug, *Pour la répopulation et contre la vie chère* (Paris, 1918), pp. 39–41.

34. John C. Hunter, "The Problem of the French Birth Rate on the Eve of World War I," *French Historical Studies* (1962), 490–503.

35. Esther Kanipe, "Working-Class Women and the Social Question in Late Nineteenth

Century France," *Proceedings of the Sixth Annual Meeting of the Western Society for French History*, 1978 (Santa Barbara, 1979), p. 302.

36. Robert Talmy, *Histoire du mouvement familiale en France, 1896–1939* (Paris, 1962), pp. 123 ff.

37. Robert Colin, "Prémices et développement de la législation familiale française," in Robert Pringent, ed., *Renouveau des idées sur la famille* (Paris, 1954), pp. 151–184.

38. Couturier, *Demain*, introduction; Deherme, *Croître*, pp. 61, 72; E. Faguet, . . . *et l'horreur des responsabilités* (Paris, 1911), p. 144; F.A. Vuillermet, *Le Suicide d'un race* (Paris, 1911), pp. 217 ff.; Ract, *Natalité*, p. 96.

39. Bertillon, *Dépopulation*, p. 240; G. Blet, *L'Avortement, est-ce un crime?* (Macon, 1921), pp. 46 ff.; M. de Roux, *L'Etat et la natalité* (Paris, 1918), pp. 83–92; Leroy-Beaulieu, *Traité*, 4:617; Louis Roya, *Les Crimes d'alcove* (Paris, 1911), pp. 26–27; Boverat, *Patriotisme*, pp. 332–336.

40. On the legislative struggle, see C. Colson, "La Tache de demain: la population," *Revue des deux mondes* 26 (1915), 840–876; C.M. Savarit, *Revue Hebdomadaire* (February 1909), pp. 242–260; Pierre Garaud and Marcel Laborde-Lacoste, *La Répression de la propagande contre la natalité* (Paris, 1921); Michel M. Raiter, *Avortement criminel et dépopulation: examen de la loi de correctionalisation* (Paris, 1925); A. Tarakdji, *L'Avortement criminel: étude médico-legale, juridique et psycho-sociale* (Paris, 1937); Guerrand, *Maternité* pp. 82 ff.; Francis Ronsin, *La Grève des ventres. Propagande néo-malthusienne et baisse de la natalité en France* (Paris, 1980), pp. 137–148.

41. See *Journal officiel: Chambre des députés* (23 July 1920), pp. 3068 ff.

42. Dyer, *Population*, pp. 63 ff.

43. See for example C. Watson, "Birth Control and Abortion in France Since 1939" *Population Studies* 5 (1951–1952), 261–264.

44. Charles Montalban, *La Petite Bible des jeunes époux* (Paris, 1885); H. de Castelnau, "De la limitation du nombre des enfants dans le mariage," *Revue de thérapeutique médico-chirurgicale* 25 (1867), 164–168; A. Corre, *La Mère et l'enfant dans les races humaines* (Paris, 1882), pp. 255–256; P. Garnier, *Onanisme seul et à deux* (Paris, 1885); P. Marrin, *Le Mariage: théorique et pratique* (Paris, 1895), pp. 283–292; Dr. Charles Féré, "Les méfaits des artifices de la fécondation," *Annales des maladies des organes génito-urinaires* 24 (1906), 811–815; and for an overview, see A.B. Liptay, *Pour et contre Malthus* (Paris 1911).

45. Dr. Henri Fischer, *De l'éducation sexuelle* (Paris, 1903); Dr. E. Toulouse, *Les Conflits intersexuels et sociaux* (Paris, 1904); Auguste Forel, *La Question sexuelle exposée aux adultes cultivés* (Paris, 1905); J. Sicard de Plauzoles, *La Fonction sexuelle* (Paris, 1908). Sicard de Plauzoles led the Société de la prophylaxie sanitaire that sought to repeal the law of 31 July 1920; see Jacques Donzelot, *The Policing of Families* (New York, 1979), p. 180.

46. For accounts of Robin's death see Giroud, *Robin*, p. 291; *Le Malthusien* (October 1912), (December 1912); *Le Gaulois* (4 September 1912), p. 2; on the movement after the war, see Humbert, *Humbert*, pp. 121–180; Job [Comte J.M.M.G. Onfroy de Bréville], *La Verité sur la question de la population* (Paris, 1924).

Index

About the Author

Angus McLaren was born in Vancouver, Canada, and did his undergraduate work at the University of British Columbia. After taking his doctorate at Harvard University, he taught at the University of Calgary and Grinnell College and was a Senior Associate Fellow at St. Antony's College, Oxford. Since 1975 he has been at the University of Victoria, where he is currently Associate Professor of History. His first book, *Birth Control in Nineteenth-Century England,* appeared in 1978. At the moment, he is writing a history of reproductive rituals in early modern Europe.